WD

A DICTIONARY OF

Sports Injuries and Disorders

A DICTIONARY OF

Sports Injuries and Disorders

O. Potparic and J. Gibson

The Parthenon Publishing Group
International Publishers in Medicine, Science & Technology

NEW YORK   LONDON

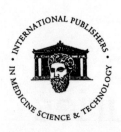

Published in the UK and Europe by
The Parthenon Publishing Group Ltd
Casterton Hall
Carnforth, Lancs, LA6 2LA, England, UK

Published in North America by
The Parthenon Publishing Group Inc.
One Blue Hill Plaza, PO Box 1564
Pearl River
New York 10965, USA

Copyright © 1996 The Parthenon Publishing Group Ltd

British Library Cataloguing in Publication Data
Potparic, O.
    Dictionary of Sports Injuries and
    Disorders
    I. Title II. Gibson, John
    617.1027

    ISBN 1-85070-686-7

Library of Congress Cataloging-in-Publication Data
Potparic, O. (Olivera)
    A dictionary of sports injuries and disorders/O. Potparic and
J. Gibson.
        p.   cm.
    ISBN 1-85070-686-7
    1. Sports medicine – Dictionaries.   2. Sports injuries –
Dictionaries.   I. Gibson, John, 1907–   . II. Title.
    [DNLM: 1. Sports Medicine – dictionaries.   2. Athletic Injuries –
dictionaries.   QT 13 P864d 1995]
RC1206.P68   1995
617.1′027′03 – dc20
DNLM/DLC
for Library of Congress   95-39884
                                                                  CIP

Typeset by Blackpool Typesetting Services Ltd.,
Blackpool, Lancashire, UK
Printed and bound by Bookcraft (Bath) Ltd., UK

Introduction

Injuries can occur in any sport. They may be mild or severe, short-lived or lifelong, and sometimes can be fatal. They can occur in beginners and experienced athletes, in amateurs and professionals. Some can be prevented by proper training, muscle strength development, co-ordination development, warm up before competing, a healthy diet and appropriate equipment and footwear. It is hoped that this book will help doctors, medical students, physiotherapists, nurses, managers, coaches and the athletes themselves.

The authors wish to thank Dr H. C. Burry of North Canterbury, New Zealand, for his information of the ugly parent syndrome.

5

Abductor digiti quinti (minimi) nerve entrapment

Entrapment in the heel of the nerve to abductor digiti quinti, which is a branch of the lateral plantar nerve, is thought to be the cause of a dull pain in the heel. Treatment is either conservative using non-steroidal anti-inflammatory drugs and local steroid injection or by surgery.

Abstinence syndrome

Other name Withdrawal syndrome

Abstinence syndrome occurs in athletes who have given up training completely after a long period of intensive training. Clinical features are anxiety, irritability, restlessness, fatigue, muscle twitching, sleep disturbances and feelings of guilt.

Achilles tendonitis

Achilles tendonitis is an inflammation of the Achilles tendon and associated paratenon (the fatty areolar tissue filling its fascial compartment). Acute tendonitis can occur in running and other activities. The patient complains of pain in the tendon and stiffness in it on getting out of bed. Clinical features are a thick edematous and tender tendon and sometimes crepitus. Treatment involves rest, non-steroidal anti-inflammatory drugs, deep pressure massage when acute symptoms have subsided, ultrasound, stretching of gastrocnemius and soleus, mobilization of the ankle and subtalar joints, and a slow return to activity.

Chronic paratenon thickening can be a complication of acute tendonitis or be a result of continued activity after symptoms have appeared. Movements of the tendon are restricted by thickening of the paratenon and its adherence to the tendon. Recurrent attacks of acute tendonitis are likely.

Achilles tendon rupture

Rupture of the Achilles tendon can be partial or complete.

Partial rupture usually occurs in runners. The patient complains of sudden sharp pain in the tendon 2–3 cm above its insertion. The pain gradually becomes milder and chronic. Clinical examination may reveal a small tender lump at the spot or a gap in the tendon. Treatment is by immobilization in plaster with the foot in plantar flexion. If this is unsuccessful, surgical treatment is necessary.

Complete rupture can occur in skiing when the skier falls forward with the foot fixed in the ski and the ankle dorsiflexed, and in rackets, basketball, running, jogging and jumping when the tendon is overflexed. Risk factors are increasing age, gout and a previous injection of corticosteroid into the tendon. It can occur in young, healthy, vigorous athletes. The patient feels a sudden snap and acute pain in the tendon and is likely to fall. Walking is difficult and with a limp. Clinical features are a visible and palpable gap in the tendon, followed by bruising and swelling. Treatment in older patients involves immobilization, but if this fails or the patient is young surgery is necessary.

Acromioclavicular joint dysfunction

Acromioclavicular joint dysfunction can be due to instability, snapping from a torn acromioclavicular cartilage, or to cystic degeneration or osteolysis at the distal end of the clavicle. It can occur in baseball pitchers and throwers. Clinical features are instability of the joint, snapping or discomfort. Treatment involves rest or surgery.

Acromioclavicular joint injury

Acromioclavicular joint injury can be due to a direct lateral blow to the shoulder or to a fall onto the outstretched hand or the outer side of the shoulder. It can occur in footballers, wrestlers, ice hockey players, cyclists and horse riders. The force of the blow is transmitted through the glenoid cavity to the acromioclavicular ligament and the coracoclavicular ligament.

First degree injury is a tear of the fibres of the acromioclavicular ligament, with pain, tenderness and swelling over the joint.

Second degree injury is a subluxation of the acromioclavicular joint due to this tearing; the clavicle is moved slightly upwards, and abduction of the arm beyond 80° can be painful for 7–10 days.

Third degree injury is a disruption of the ligaments stabilizing the acromioclavicular joint and of the attachments of the deltoid and trapezius muscles to the clavicle, which is displaced upwards; the patient complains of severe pain.

Treatment of first degree injury involves a reduction of shoulder movements, ice and analgesics. Treatment of second degree injury is by rest, supporting the arm in a sling, analgesics and, if pain continues, by the injection of a local anesthetic and corticosteroid. Treatment of third degree injury is conservative at first and surgical if this is not effective.

Acromioclavicular joint meniscus injury

Injury to the acromioclavicular meniscus can cause recurrent attacks of a painful catching sensation on moving the shoulder. Surgical removal of the disc may be necessary.

Acromioclavicular joint osteoarthritis

Acromioclavicular joint osteoarthritis can be due to earlier trauma or to rupture of the rotator cuff with subluxation of the head of the humerus upwards. It can be asymptomatic or cause pain, especially when the arm is swung above the head. Pain and crepitus are produced by passive movement of the joint. Treatment involves rest, analgesic drugs, injection of local anesthetic and corticosteroid, and mobilization techniques.

Acromioclavicular joint overuse

Acromioclavicular joint overuse is manifested by a dull ache in the joint and sometimes distal clavicular osteolysis. It is the result of multiple microtrauma. It can be a result of strength-training exercises in weight-lifters and others. Treatment involves rest and non-steroidal anti-inflammatory drugs.

Acute anterior cervical spinal cord injury syndrome

Acute anterior cervical spinal cord injury syndrome is the result of a severe injury to the neck that can occur in contact sports such as American football and rugby. It is characterized by an immediate acute paralysis of all four limbs with loss of pain and temperature up to the level of the lesion, but with preservation of the posterior column sensations of position, motion, vibration and light touch.

Acute brachial neuropathy
See Parsonage–Turner syndrome

Acute brachial plexus stretch injury

Acute brachial plexus stretch injury is due to a blow which tilts the head and neck to the opposite side with depression of the shoulder. The brachial plexus is excessively stretched. Clinical features are a burning pain radiating from the shoulder to the hand, lasting for a few seconds, followed by weakness of the arm and hand lasting for 1–2 min. If recovery does not take place in that time, the cervical spine and brachial plexus have probably been severely injured. Treatment is by wearing a sling and not taking part in any sport or athletics. Recovery in 3–4 months is likely in 90% of cases.

Acute cervical radiculopathy

Acute cervical radiculopathy can occur in weight-lifters. It is characterized by neck and shoulder pain and pain radiating down the arm. Treatment is conservative. Structural degeneration of cervical vertebrae may be demonstrated by X-ray and magnetic resonance imaging and this is a contraindication to resuming the sport.

Acute cervical sprain or strain

Acute cervical sprain and strain can occur in wrestlers. A sprain is usually due to a hyperextensive twist of the neck. A strain is a tear of one of the neck muscles. Symptoms are similar for the two types of injury, with pain, tenderness and localized inhibition of contraction of the injured muscle. With a sprain the pain may not appear until the next day and can cease after a few minutes with the return of full muscle function. With a strain muscle movements can produce more severe pain. Treatment involves immobilization in a collar, ice and non-steroidal anti-inflammatory drugs, followed by isometric exercises.

Acute mountain sickness
See High altitude disorders

Adduction muscle strain or rupture

Adduction muscle strain and rupture are due to a sudden forceful contraction of the muscles when the hip is abducted and the thigh is externally rotated. A strain may present with a mild but gradually worsening pain, and a severe strain presents with sudden pain in the groin or middle of the thigh. Clinical features are an area of tenderness, pain made worse by passive abduction and by a defect or palpable mass when the muscle ruptures. Treatment involves rest, ice, compression, elevation of the limb and non-steroidal anti-inflammatory drugs, followed by stretching and strengthening exercises and a gradual return to sporting activities.

Adductor canal syndrome

Adductor canal syndrome is a rare disorder which can occur in young athletes. They complain of lower leg claudication made worse by exercise and relieved by rest. The femoral pulse may be weak or absent. It has been attributed to compression of the femoral artery in the adductor canal by a musculotendinous band. The saphenous nerve may also be entrapped in the canal.

Adductor longus tendonitis

Other name Rider's strain

Adductor longus tendonitis is a strain of the muscle at its tendinous origin or a few centimeters from its musculotendinous junction. The patient complains of pain in the groin, a pain which is made worse by contraction or stretching of the muscle; there is tenderness over the lesion. Treatment involves rest, non-steroidal anti-inflammatory drugs, injection of local anesthetic and corticosteroid into the musculotendinous junction, and stretching exercises in a warm pool.

Adolescent swimmer's back

Adolescent swimmer's back is pain in the back of adolescents who swim using the butterfly stroke. It can be associated with Scheuermann kyphosis (adolescent kyphosis), which can cause pain in the back, stiffness and a rounded back. Affected swimmers should use other strokes during adolescence.

Algodystrophy

Algodystrophy is characterized by pain, tenderness, vasomotor changes, loss of mobility following any injury and, in particular, a Colles' fracture of the lower end of the radius.

Amenorrhea

Amenorrhea (or oligomenorrhea when the menstrual cycle length is longer than 35 days) can occur in women athletes engaged in intensive training. Rowers, runners, gymnasts and cyclists are most likely to be affected. There is an association with low body weight, low body fat, low calorie intake, previous menstrual disturbances, psychological stress and intensity of training. The pulsatile release of gonadotropin releasing hormone is affected and the secretion of pituitary gonadotropins is reduced, with secondary ovarian failure following. Complications are osteoporosis and stress fractures. In most women athletes menstruation becomes normal when competitive stress is removed.

Anabolic steroid poisoning

Anabolic steroids can be taken by weight-lifters, wrestlers, swimmers, shot-putters and javelin throwers to increase their muscle mass. The consequence can be enlargement of the heart, sudden death from heart failure, peliosis hepatis, carcinoma of colon and kidney, and acne. Men can develop testicular atrophy, infertility, carcinoma of the prostate and outbursts of rage and violence. Women can develop total body failure, with failure of the kidneys, liver and pancreas, and also deafness, shrunken breasts, facial hair and a deep voice.

Ankle dislocation

Dislocation of the talotibial joint is uncommon without fracture because of the strength of the ligaments. The dislocation can be posterior, anterior or superior and is due to severe strain placed on the joint. Treatment is by immediate reduction. A non-weight-bearing cast is worn for 4–6 months for an incomplete tear; surgical treatment may be necessary for a complete tear.

Ankle impingement syndromes

Anterior impingement syndrome can occur in gymnasts performing tumbling routines and on bad short landings when the foot is hyperflexed. The patient complains of an intermittent ache in the front of the ankle which is tender. Treatment involves rest, ice and non-steroidal anti-inflammatory drugs.

Posterior impingement syndrome can occur in gymnasts and presents as lateral pain at the back of ankle when the os calcis closes against the posterior lip of the tibia. It can follow an ankle sprain and disruption of the ankle ligaments. An os trigonum or a long talar process at the back of the ankle are sometimes present; these processes can be fractured by trauma. Treatment involves rest and non-steroidal anti-inflammatory drugs. An os trigonum may have to be removed surgically.

Ankle instability

Ankle instability is a chronic condition which can follow any injury of an ankle ligament. It is characterized by discomfort or pain in the ankle, swelling of the ankle, stiffness and muscle weakness. The term 'functional instability' is used to describe a feeling of the joint giving way or recurrent sprains. Treatment can involve ankle taping and bracing, but if this is ineffective surgery may be necessary.

Ankle meniscoid lesions

Meniscoid lesions of the ankle can follow repeated ankle sprains and cause instability, swelling and chronic pain. The symptoms may be due to the presence of fibrous tissue or a torn fragment of the anterior talofibular ligament in the ankle joint. Treatment can be conservative or surgical.

Ankle sprains

Ankle sprains are the most frequent sports injuries. They can be a sprain of either the anterior talofibular ligament, the anterior tibiofibular ligament, the medial ligament or the posterior talofibular ligament.

Anterior talofibular ligament sprain can result from forced plantar flexion or by a sudden excessive degree of inversion.

Anterior tibiofibular ligament sprain can be due either to a forced dorsiflexion of the ankle with the anterior part of talar body forced into the joint, or to an eversion injury in which the talus is forced against the medial malleolus and fibres of the anterior tibiofibular ligament are liable to be torn. Separation of the joint can occur.

Medial ligament sprain is uncommon, as eversion injuries are unusual and the ligament is strong enough to stand up to any strain placed upon it.

Posterior talofibular sprain can occur in a long-jumper who lands on his or her feet with the ankle acutely dorsiflexed.

On spraining the ankle a patient is likely to hear an audible snap and to have pain on stretching or compressing the ligament.

Movement of the joint is also likely to cause pain. Treatment involves rest, compression, elevation, ice and non-steroidal anti-inflammatory drugs. This is followed by exercises within the limit of the pain, isokinetic and postural re-education exercises, and stretching techniques of the tissues around the ankle and of the Achilles tendon. The ankle should be strapped for practice exercises and games.

Anorexia nervosa

Anorexia nervosa can occur in girl and young women athletes, especially in gymnasts and runners (less commonly in male athletes), who, afraid of putting on weight, begin by reducing their food intake and progress to eating little or nothing. Clinical features are semi-starvation, disappearance of cutaneous fat, an obsessive pursuit of thinness, denial of illness, insistence that they are too fat in spite of evidence of gross loss of weight, disturbance of body image and amenorrhea. Associated conditions can be bulimia nervosa (binge eating), excessive consumption of water or caffeine, low blood pressure, reduced cardiac output, anemia, leukopenia, hypoglycemia, infections, and osteoporosis leading to stress fractures and compression fracture of vertebral bodies. About 40% recover. Others may remain chronically ill with a likelihood of periodic exacerbations. Death can be due to inanition, electrolyte disturbance, infection or suicide.

Anterior drawer test of the ankle

Anterior drawer test of the ankle is a test of ankle instability. The patient must be relaxed. The test is performed by direct pressure from behind the heel with the foot in plantar flexion. The examiner stabilizes the tibia by grasping the leg just above the ankle with one hand and attempts to move the foot forward by pressure on the heel. The normal movement forward is less than 5 mm. More than this suggests ankle instability. The affected ankle should be compared with the unaffected one because of anatomical variations.

Anterior drawer test of the knee

Anterior drawer test of the knee is a test of knee instability due to ligament injury. The patient lies supine with the hip flexed to 45° and the knee to 90°. The examiner sits on the patient's foot in order to stabilize it, feels the hamstring tendons to ensure that they are relaxed, and then grasps the upper end of the tibia and pushes it to and fro to ascertain the degree of anterior movement. An excessive degree of movement suggests a rupture of the anterior cruciate ligament, but the test is sometimes negative with a ruptured ligament. The test can be positive with tears of the medial and lateral ligaments of the knee.

See also Knee anterior cruciate ligament injury, posterior drawer test of the knee

Anterior glenohumeral subluxation

Anterior glenohumeral subluxation can occur in wrestlers. Clinical features are likely to be a feeling of the shoulder slipping in and out, pain anteriorly and/or posteriorly tenderness on palpation and a decrease in the range of muscle movements. Treatment of an acute subluxation involves the use a sling and swathe for 2–3 weeks, followed by strengthening exercises.

Anterior inferior iliac spine avulsion

Avulsion of the anterior inferior iliac spine can be due to spasm of rectus femoris in adolescent players of American football before they have reached full skeletal maturity. Clinical features are pain and spasm. Treatment involves rest and positioning to relax rectus femoris until symptom-free, and then a gradual return to full activity. Non-union is a complication which may require surgical excision of the spine portion which is not united.

Anterior interosseous syndrome

Anterior interosseous syndrome is paralysis of flexor pollicis longus and index profundus, either alone or together, associated with pain for 24 hours. It can occur in weight-lifters and gymnasts. Treatment involves rest and non-steroidal anti-inflammatory drugs or corticosteroids.

Anterior shoulder pain syndrome

Anterior shoulder pain syndrome is a sprain of the supraspinatus and subscapularis muscles and of the middle and inferior glenohumeral ligaments of the shoulder capsule in baseball pitchers as a result of faulty technique. The clinical feature is anterior joint line pain usually experienced in the late cocking/ early acceleration phase. Treatment involves rest from pitching and other activities aggravating the condition, and by rotator cuff strengthening exercises.

Anterior superior iliac spine avulsion

Avulsion of the anterior superior iliac spine can occur in adolescent athletes while it is still attached to the pelvis by cartilage. It is due to a sudden pull by the sartorius muscle. The patient complains of a sudden sharp pain in the anterior region of the pelvis, a pain which is reproduced by forced extension of the hip while the knee is flexed. The athlete can walk but not run. The site is swollen and tender. The diagnosis is confirmed by X-ray. Treatment is conservative, involving bed rest for 3 weeks with immobilization of the leg, and this is followed by walking on crutches for 4–6 weeks. Surgical treatment is sometimes necessary for severely displaced fragments.

Anterior talotibial impingement
See Athlete's ankle

Anterior tarsal syndrome

Other name Deep peroneal nerve entrapment

Anterior tarsal syndrome is due to entrapment of the deep peroneal nerve beneath the inferior retinaculum at the ankle. The patient is likely to complain of numbness or slight pain in the dorsomedial aspect of the foot radiating sometimes into the first web space. Wearing a loose shoe or padding may relieve the symptoms, but if this is ineffective surgical treatment is necessary.

Anterior thigh compartment syndrome

Anterior thigh compartment syndrome can follow a blunt blow to the front of the thigh. In an athlete with a blood dyscrasia the blow need only be a slight one. Hemorrhage into the compartment is followed by inflammation. Clinical features are pain, tenderness and swelling in the front of the thigh. Other features can be effusion into the knee joint as well as paresthesiae in the front of the thigh and the medial aspect of the leg and foot. With a severe and inadequately treated hemorrhage complications can be gross loss of muscle and myositis ossificans. If the condition is acute an immediate fasciotomy is necessary. Mild symptoms are treated with rest, ice and elevation of the limb. With graduated exercises the patient should be able to engage in full activities in a few weeks, but in contact sports he or she should wear a thigh pad.

See also Compartment syndromes of the leg

Aortic rupture

Traumatic rupture of the thoracic aorta can occur when an athlete travelling at high speed crashes into an immobile obstacle, as can happen in skiing, water-skiing and sky-diving. Complete rupture causes immediate death, but with a partial rupture the patient may survive long enough to undergo surgery.

See also Sudden death in athletes

Appendicitis

Acute appendicitis has occurred to athletes undergoing intensive training.

Apprehension test
See Patellar dislocation

Asthma

Asthma attacks due to bronchial constriction can be induced by exercise. The athlete may have noticed previously that he or she wheezes or coughs after exercise. The attack may occur during the exercise, within 15 minutes of stopping it, and sometimes several hours later. It can occur in middle-distance and long-distance runners due to the inhalation of aeroallergens and in skiers due to the inhalation of cold air. Prevention is by physical training, avoiding running in the open air and outdoor exercise in cold weather, avoidance of any sport known to bring on an attack, warming up before exercise, and the use of antiasthmatic drugs such as sodium cromoglycate (but due regard should be paid in competitions to the rules of regulating bodies such as the International Olympic Committee).

17

Athlete's ankle

Other name Anterior talotibial impingement

Athlete's ankle is pain, swelling and discomfort in the ankle due to entrapment of soft tissue or a bony outgrowth between the anterior aspect of the tibia and the talus during dorsiflexion of the ankle. It is likely to occur in football players, soccer players and ballet dancers who are called to perform extremes of dorsiflexion, sudden acceleration and jumping. It can progress to talotibial exostoses. Treatment may be conservative at first, but surgery is likely to be necessary.

See also Talotibial exostoses

Athlete's foot

Other name Tinea pedis

Athlete's foot is a fungal infection due to *Trichophyton, Microsporum* or *Epidermophyton*. It presents as red, very itchy, scaly areas between the toes and on the soles of the feet. A fissure in a toe web can be very painful. Prevention is by cleanliness and good foot care. An infected athlete should not share a communal bath, should be last under a shower, should not walk with bare feet on surfaces walked on by others and should have his/her own towel. Treatment involves the use of imidazole powder.

Auricular hematoma

Auricular hematoma is a common injury in wrestling and boxing. Treatment of an acute hematoma involves needle aspiration and a pressure dressing. Failure to treat can result in a 'cauliflower ear'.

Avalanche deaths

Many skiers are killed in avalanches every year – about 150 in the European Alps. The chances of survival are high (92%) in the first 15 minutes and drop sharply to 30% after 35 minutes. Rescue depends on the action of other skiers present, so all skiers should learn techniques for finding, rescuing and resuscitating victims.

Axillary artery injury

The axillary artery can be injured by fractures of the clavicle, the neck of the humerus and the neck of the scapula, and by dislocation of the shoulder. The clinical feature is a diminished pulse in the arm, with or without temperature loss and color decrease. Investigation is by angiogram. Treatment involves vascular repair and care of the injury causing the arterial lesion.

Axillary artery occlusion

Axillary artery occlusion can occur in throwers such as baseball pitchers. Transient occlusion may be due to irritation by the outstretched pectoralis minor muscle, and repeated trauma can cause arterial damage and thrombosis. Clinical features are pain and tenderness over the supraclavicular space, diminished or absent pulses in the arm, cyanosis, decreased skin temperature and claudication. The diagnosis can be confirmed by arteriogram. Treatment is surgical and involves either a thrombectomy or sympathectomy.

Axillary nerve injury

Axillary nerve injury can occur in American football, rugby, gymnastics, wrestling and mountaineering. It can be caused by a blow to the shoulder, dislocation of the shoulder or fracture of the proximal humerus when stretching of the nerve occurs. Clinical features are weakness in elevation and abduction of the arm, with or without numbness in the lateral aspect of the upper arm, and wasting of the deltoid muscle. Treatment of a partial injury involves rest, a sling and physiotherapy. Recovery can be expected within 3 months. Surgical intervention is necessary if there is no improvement after 3–4 months and for severe injury.

Axillary vein thrombosis
See Effort thrombosis

B

Backpack palsy

Backpack palsy is a compression injury to the nerves around the shoulder. The nerves compressed can be the long thoracic, the suprascapular and the spinal accessory. Clinical features are weakness of the shoulder and arm, atrophy of shoulder girdle muscles and winging of the scapula. Treatment involves not carrying a backpack for some time and then modifying carrying methods.

Baseball finger
See Mallet finger

Bennett's fracture

Bennett's fracture is a fracture/dislocation of the first metacarpal bone; a small volar lip is detached and the shaft is subluxated dorsally by abductor pollicis longus. Treatment is surgical.

Biceps brachii avulsion

Avulsion of the biceps brachii tendon at the elbow can occur in weight-lifters. The patient feels a tearing or popping sensation and pain and presents with bruising, swelling and tenderness in the antecubital fossa. Treatment is surgical.

Biceps tendon rupture

Biceps tendon rupture can occur in gymnasts and throwers. Clinical features are a sudden snap, a sharp pain and the appearance of a gap in the muscle. Treatment involves ice and a sling. The rupture can heal but there is likely to be permanent weakness in the muscle. Surgical repair is sometimes necessary.

Bicipital tendonitis

Bicipital tendonitis can follow the overuse of shoulder movements and may be associated with chronic or recurrent tenosynovitis of the investing synovial sheath. Damage to the superior labrum of the glenoid fossa can be associated with avulsion of the tendinous attachment to the labrum (SLAP syndrome). Clinical features are pain over the shoulder joint and radiating down the arm, as well as pain on shoulder movement or on stretching the tendon. Treatment involves rest, nonsteroidal anti-inflammatory drugs, passive movements and injection of local anesthetic and corticosteroid into the site of maximal tenderness. If the response is inadequate, or if the tendonitis recurs, surgery is necessary.

Big toe fractures

Big toe fractures can be either a stress fracture of the proximal phalanx or a fracture of a sesamoid bone.

Stress fracture of the proximal phalanx is most likely to occur in an athlete with a hallux valgus deformity and to be an avulsion fracture. Clinical features are pain, tenderness and reduced mobility of the metacarpophalangeal joint. Treatment involves rest from athletic activities and taping the toe.

Sesamoid fracture is usually in the medial sesamoid and is characterized by medial plantar pain and edema. Treatment involves rest and a foam-padding orthesis. Surgical excision may be necessary if the fracture does not heal.

Blisters

Blisters can occur on the feet of athletes due to friction between the skin and a shoe, especially in environments of heat and humidity; they can also appear on the hands of gymnasts and rowers. Preventive measures include hardening the skin with tannic acid (10% solution) and wearing two pairs of powdered socks. Treatment involves draining the blister with a sterile needle and covering with occlusive tape. Infection of a blister can be a complication.

Blood doping

Blood doping is a blood transfusion given to an athlete just before an athletic event to increase his or her oxygen capacity and so enhance his or her performance. The athlete could become infected with HIV if the blood used in the transfusion is contaminated with the virus.

Boutonnière deformity

Boutonnière deformity is due to disruption of the central extensor tendon slip at its insertion into the middle phalanx and is associated with tearing of the triangular ligament on the dorsum of the middle phalanx. There may be an avulsion fracture from the dorsum of the base of the middle phalanx. The deformity is a flexion deformity of the proximal interphalangeal joint. Treatment of an immediate injury involves splinting the proximal interphalangeal joint in full extension for 6 weeks and passive stretching of the distal phalangeal joint into flexion. However, many athletes do not present for treatment until the end of a season and a neglected deformity is more difficult to treat, especially if contractures have developed; the choice is between surgery and the acceptance by the patient of a permanent deformity.

Bowler's thumb

Bowler's thumb can occur in those who play ten-pin bowling. In bowling the edge of the thumb-hold is pressed against the palmar aspect of the proximal phalanx of the thumb, compressing the digital nerves against the sheath of flexor pollicis longus. In time a neuroma can develop in one of the nerves. Clinical features are pain in the palmar aspect of the thumb of the bowling hand, numbness in the thumb pulp and a nodule. The nodule presents as a firm swelling over the proximal phalanx of the thumb that can be moved transversely but not longitudinally. Treatment involves ceasing to play ten-pin bowling and excision of the neuroma.

Boxing injuries

Boxing injuries are common. Severe injuries are more likely to be suffered by professional boxers than by amateurs. They can be due to falls onto the floor as well as to blows from an opponent.

Concussion can cause headache, nausea, dizziness, speech disturbances, extrapyramidal disturbances and lack of co-ordination.

Facial injuries can be lacerations (inside and outside the mouth), cut lips, nasal bone fracture, jaw fracture and injury to the bony rim and floor of the orbit.

See also Facial laceration, subchondral hematoma of the ear; zygomal fracture

Eye injuries can be lid lacerations and ecchymoses, corneal abrasion and scarring, choroidal tears and hemorrhages, choroidoretinal atrophy and pigmentation, cataract, lens subluxation, angle recession, retinal edema, atrophic retinal holes and retinal detachment.

Temporomandibular injuries can be alveolar fracture and tooth avulsion.

Head injuries can be a subdural hematoma (due to rapid deceleration when the head strikes the floor), an epidural hematoma, a subarachnoid hemorrhage and fracture of the skull.

Hand injuries can be 'boxer's knuckle' (any metacarpophalangeal joint injury), traumatic bossing (bony hypertrophy at the metacarpophalangeal joints), disruption of the extensor mechanism of the metacarpophalangeal joint, fracture of a metacarpal neck, carpometacarpal joint dislocation and fracture/dislocation of the thumb.

Chronic neurological injury (dementia pugilistica).
See Punch-drunk syndrome

Brachial plexus injury

Brachial plexus injury can be due to a blow to the shoulder girdle of the involved side with the head and neck laterally flexed away from the site of injury or, less commonly, with the head laterally flexed towards the same side of the injury due to a forced hyperextension of the head and neck. It is classified as either grade I – a reversible aberration in axonal function with resolution immediately or within 2 weeks; grade II – disruption of the axon and myelin sheath with intact epineurium, and wallerian degeneration spreading distally from the point of injury (for function to return complete regeneration must occur); or grade III – severe laceration, stretching or crushing with disruption of endoneurium, epineurium and perineurium.

With a grade I injury the athlete complains of a sharp burning feeling (a 'burner' or 'stinger') in the neck that radiates to the shoulder and down the arm to the hand, paresthesiae in the arm, and weakness of shoulder abduction, elbow flexion and external humeral rotation. There is a full pain-free range of neck movements. Recovery takes place quickly. With a grade II injury the athlete complains of similar symptoms and biceps weakness, but recovery is delayed for 3–4 weeks and may not be complete for 6 months. A grade III injury is uncommon in athletes in the absence of a perforating injury or dislocation of the shoulder. Recovery may take a year or more, and the athlete should be advised not to risk a second injury and to take up a sport in which it is not likely to occur. Measures to prevent recurrence include neck and shoulder strengthening exercises and wearing a horse-collar neck roll.

Brachial plexus neuropathy
See Parsonage–Turner syndrome

Brain swelling

Brain swelling can occur after any brain injury and without edema of the brain; it is thought to be due to an increase in cerebral blood volume. The swelling can be localized following a focal injury, but it is generalized after a generalized injury. It can occur minutes or hours after the injury, or there may not be a serious rise of intracranial pressure for several days. A localized swelling may not have serious consequences. The usual clinical presentation of a generalized swelling is that of temporary recovery from the initial injury followed some time later by a lapse into coma.

Breaststroke swimmer's knee

Breaststroke swimmer's knee presents as pain and inflammation in the upper attachment of the medial collateral ligament of the knee due to the stress placed on the ligament by the action of the legs in the breaststroke. Nowadays it is rare as the kick in the stroke is narrower. Treatment is by rest and ultrasound.

Bronchospasm

Exercise-induced bronchospasm can occur in 3–10% of athletes. It is likely to occur in those with a history of asthma or allergic rhinitis. Clinical features are shortness of breath, tightness of breathing, coughing or wheezing lasting for 5–15 min after exercise and sometimes reappearing 3–6 hours later. It is not a contraindication to participation in sport provided that medical advice is followed on prevention and treatment.

Bunionette

Other name Tailor's bunion

Bunionette is a prominence on the lateral eminence of the fifth metatarsal head (said to be produced in tailors who sat cross-legged). It can be associated with hallux valgus deformity. Pressure by footwear can produce irritation, pain and swelling by pressing on a bursa over it, and the bursa can become inflamed. Treatment is either conservative by wearing different footwear and padding, or surgical.

Burners

Burners is the name given by players of American football to a burning pain radiating down the arm. Other features are transient paresthesiae and weakness of the deltoid muscle. It is thought to be due to neuropraxia of the brachial plexus. It can last for short time, for weeks, or for a year or more. Treatment involves rest and wearing a neck collar until free from symptoms. Recurrence is common.

Burnout

Other name Overtraining syndrome

Burnout can occur in athletes who train for too long and too fiercely and in top athletes after losing; it leaves them feeling that they have not achieved their ambitions. Clinical features are likely to be depression, tension, fatigue, anger, reduction in performance, painful muscles and sore throat. There is a strong psychological component. Physical findings and laboratory studies are normal. Treatment is by stopping training and psychotherapy.

See also Overuse injuries

Bushke's disease

Bushke's disease is osteochondrosis of the cuneiform bone, which can occur in young athletes. They present with pain in the midfoot. Treatment involves rest and a mid-tarsal support.

Butland's test

Butland's test is a measure of exercise tolerance in which the subject is asked to walk at his own pace at a constant speed on a level surface, and the distance covered in 2 minutes and 6 minutes are measured. It is a modification of McGavin's test, in which the patient is asked to walk for 12 minutes.

C

Calcaneal apophysitis
See Sever's disease

Calcaneal fracture

An avulsion fracture of the anterior process of the calcaneus can occur in severe injuries of the foot with the bifurcate ligament (the calcaneocuboid and calcaneonavicular ligaments) playing a part in the avulsion but remaining intact. The fracture may be displaced or undisplaced. Clinical features are pain and tenderness at the site. Conservative treatment involves immobilization by wraps or a non-weight-bearing cast with a gradual return to full weight-bearing. A pseudoarthrosis can be treated with the injection of a local anesthetic. Surgical excision of the fragment may be required if these measures fail.

Calcaneal osteochondritis

Osteochondritis of the calcaneus occurs mainly in boys aged 7–14 years who are engaged in sports such as athletics and football in which there is a large amount of running. A contributory factor can be a valgus hindfoot deformity with inefficiency of the Achilles tendon and a reduction of passive ankle dorsiflexion. Traction by the tendon on the un-united calcaneal apophysis causes pain in the heel and stiffness. At the insertion of the tendon there is thickening, swelling and tenderness. An X-ray may show sclerosis and fragmentation of the apophysis. Treatment involves rest and a pad to raise the heel.

Calcaneodynia
See Heel pain

Camel racing injury

Camel racing jockeys in the Near East are boys aged 10–11 years who are liable to sustain a spiral fracture of the middle to lower third of the fibula owing to congestion at the start of a race. It can be prevented by wearing protective pads.

Capitate fracture

Capitate fracture can be due to a direct blow or to forced palmar or dorsiflexion. Clinical features are pain, tenderness and swelling over the fracture. Complications are avascular necrosis, an associated fracture of the scaphoid and perilunate dislocation. Treatment of a non-displaced fracture involves immobilization in a short arm cast for 6 weeks. A displaced fracture requires surgical pinning.

Capitate osteochondrosis

Osteochondrosis of the capitate can occur in gymnasts, probably as a result of microtrauma. Clinical features are pain, tenderness and swelling over the bone, as well as a decrease of grip strength. The bone shows avascular necrosis with absorption of bone and sclerosis. Treatment may require partial resection.

Capitellar osteochondritis dissecans

Osteochondritis dissecans of the capitellum can occur in adolescent baseball pitchers. Clinical features are a gradual onset of pain in the elbow, followed by stiffness, restriction of movement, swelling and clicking or grinding. An X-ray is likely to show decalcification and cysts. Treatment involves taking a permanent rest from pitching, passive stretching exercises and surgery for loose bodies and for a large osteochondral defect.

Carpal tunnel syndrome

Carpal tunnel syndrome is due to compression of the median nerve in the carpal tunnel, which is formed by the transverse carpal ligament in front and by the carpal bones at the sides and behind. The compression is usually due to flexor tenosynovitis within the tunnel, which in athletes is a result of repetitive grasping and flexion movements. Clinical features are tingling, burning and weakness in the thumb, index finger and lateral half of the middle finger, with wasting of the opponens pollicis and abductor pollicis brevis muscles when the compression is severe. Treatment involves splinting, non-steroidal anti-inflammatory drugs and corticosteroid injection into the canal.

Cauliflower ear
See Subchondral hematoma of the ear

Cephalalgia
See Exertional headache

Cervical intervertebral disc injury

Cervical intervertebral disc injury can be a herniation of the disc with neurological evidence of pressure on the cervical cord. It can result from a head impact in contact sports. Acute rupture of a disc may lead to quadriplegia. Intervertebral disc narrowing and marginal osteophytes can be due to the repetitive loading of head impacts in American football.

Cervical sprain syndrome

Cervical sprain syndrome can follow a collision in contact sports. The patient complains that his or her neck has jammed, together with pain and limitation of movement in the neck. No abnormalities are found on neurological examination and X-ray. Treatment involves immobilization with a soft collar, analgesics and non-steroidal anti-inflammatory drugs.

Cervicospinal fractures

Fractures of the cervical spine can occur in football, trampoline and water sports.

Fracture of C1 can be (a) a posterior arch fracture, which is the most common; or (b) a burst fracture of the ring from direct compression of the cervical spine. The latter is not usually associated with a neurological injury.

Fracture of C2 is usually a fracture of the odontoid process through either the tip at the attachment of the alar ligaments, the base, the body or the pedicles. The first of these is a rare and stable lesion, while the second requires surgical treatment and the third is treated with immobilization. Fracture of the pedicles may cause a spinal cord injury which can vary from slight to severe. Os odontoideum is a congenital condition in which the odontoid process has not fused with the body of the cervical vertebra and it can be mistaken for a fracture. This condition increases the risk of sustaining a C2 fracture, so any person with it should not engage in contact sports.

Fractures of C3–C7 are usually compression fractures of the vertebral body and can be associated with neurological lesions which vary from slight to severe (e.g. quadriplegia).

Cervicospinal subluxation

Subluxation of cervical vertebrae can occur in contact sports such as American football and rugby as a result of an axial compression fracture. An X-ray is likely to show narrowing of the intervertebral discs, anterior angulation and displacement of the vertebral bodies, and fanning of the vertebral spines. There are no neurological abnormalities associated with this injury. The posterior structures of the spine may be disrupted with marked instability.

Charley horse
See Quadriceps muscle contusion

Chin–sternum–heart syndrome

Chin–sternum–heart syndrome can occur when a parachute jumper with a partially opened parachute makes a hard upright landing. His chin strikes the sternum and the sternum strikes the heart. Contusion of the heart can occur. It may be asymptomatic or present with precordial pain (similar to that produced by myocardial infarction), palpitations, tachycardia, rhythm disturbances, heart murmurs and pericardial friction rub.

Chondromalacia patellae
See Patellofemoral pain syndrome

Chronic overuse tendonitis

Chronic overuse tendonitis is due to repetitive minimal loading of a tendon, causing degeneration and diminished blood supply in the tendon and inflammatory changes in surrounding tissues. It is likely to occur in the supraspinatus tendon in weight-lifters, javelin and discus throwers, and swimmers, in the adductor pollicis longus and extensor pollicis brevis tendon in rowers, in the patellar tendon in jumpers and in the Achilles tendon in runners. Rupture of the tendon can happen spontaneously. Spontaneous recovery from tendonitis can occur. Treatment involves rest, non-steroidal anti-inflammatory drugs, cortico-steroid injection and therapeutic exercises. Surgical treatment is required for rupture.

Clavicular fracture

Fractures of the clavicle can be due to a fall on an outstretched arm or to a blow from a hockey or lacrosse stick. The patient complains of pain at the site of the fracture and supports his/her arm, which unsupported droops downwards and forwards. The fracture may be at either the middle third, the medial third, the lateral third, the acromioclavicular joint or the sternoclavicular joint. Treatment is by support, reduction, or open or closed reduction with internal fixation. The fracture is likely to heal in 4–6 weeks in young athletes and in 6 weeks or more in older athletes. Non-union can be a complication and will require surgical treatment with internal fixation or bone grafting. A return to non-contact sports should not take place until the fracture is completely healed. A return to contact sports should be delayed for 4–6 months.

Clavicular osteolysis

Osteolysis of the clavicle is a loss of calcium as a result of multiple microtrauma from falls on to the shoulder by judo sportsmen and cyclists, in weight-lifters and athletes who have included weight-lifting in their training, and by shoulder contact in American football, ice hockey, field hockey and rugby. It can follow acromioclavicular dislocation. It is uncommon in female athletes, in whom it does not result from microtrauma. The patient is likely to complain of pain which restricts movement of the shoulder and there may be tenderness and deformity of the acromioclavicular joint. The diagnosis is made by X-ray, which is likely to show osteoporosis, loss of subchondral bony detail and cystic changes in the distal end of the clavicle. The disorder may be self-limiting with a duration of 1–2 years. Treatment involves rest from any activities that promote the condition and non-steroidal anti-inflammatory drugs. Excision of the lateral end of the clavicle may become necessary.

Coach's finger

Coach's finger is a dorsal dislocation of a proximal interphalangeal joint due to being struck by a ball. The injury usually occurs at the proximal interphalangeal joint, with the middle phalanx being subluxated by the pull of the extensor tendon. It has acquired its name from the advice often given by a coach to the sportsman or woman to continue playing, advice which is likely to cause deterioration of the joint. Treatment of a closed injury can be non-operative, but surgical treatment is sometimes necessary. If an open injury is untreated the consequences can be serious.

Coccygeal fracture

Coccygeal fracture is produced by a fall in a sitting position or by a kick. It is common when a rider falls from a horse. The patient complains of pain and tenderness. Diagnosis is confirmed by X-ray. Treatment involves rest and ice. Padding should be worn when the patient returns to sporting activities. Surgical removal of the bone may be necessary for the rare case in which the fracture does not heal and continues to cause pain and disability.

Common peroneal nerve entrapment

In runners, entrapment of the common peroneal nerve at the edge of the origin of peroneus longus muscle can cause pain and numbness throughout the distribution of the nerve.

Compartment syndromes of the leg

Compartment syndromes of the leg below the knee are due to a rise in tissue pressure, reduced capillary blood perfusion, and muscle edema and ischemia in the anterior, superficial posterior, deep posterior and lateral compartments which are enclosed within layers of deep fascia. They can result from the fracture of the tibia, a crush injury, the rupture of a muscle, a circumferential burn or a plaster cast. Runners are the athletes who most frequently develop this problem.

An *acute compartment syndrome* can occur in people who have just started running and have overexerted themselves, or it can be due to one of the causes mentioned above. It is characterized by the sudden onset of very acute pain in the muscle, inability to continue running and sometimes a patch of warm edematous skin over the muscle. The patient should be admitted to hospital immediately for an emergency fasciotomy to enable the muscle to bulge through the incision and so decompress the compartment. If this is not performed quickly, necrosis of muscle as well as motor and sensory loss will take place and the patient will have a permanent disability.

Chronic compartment syndrome is less definite and may persist in a mild form for several years before treatment is sought. The pathophysiology is unclear. The intracompartmental pressure is raised and the rise is increased during exercise. A runner is likely to complain that he or she is free from pain during the 'off season', and that it gradually develops as he or she starts training and persists when he or she stops his or her activities. Treatment is by fasciotomy.

See also Anterior thigh compartment syndrome

Concussion

Concussion is a reversible pathophysiological disorder of cerebral function without evidence of structural damage to the brain. It can be caused by either a blow to the head, a fall on to the head, or a forceful blow to the body that results in a sudden acceleration–deceleration of the brain within the skull. It can be mild, moderate or severe.

Mild concussion (grade I) presents with confusion and disorientation lasting for a few moments, with a dazed look and some lack of co-ordination in gait. There is no amnesia and complete recovery occurs within 5–15 minutes. The athlete may return to sporting events that day after complete recovery.

Moderate concussion (grade II) presents with confusion, disorientation, lack of co-ordination, post-traumatic amnesia and the development of retrograde amnesia 5–10 minutes later. The athlete should not return to sporting events for at least 1 week and only then when recovery is complete. He can develop a postconcussional syndrome at a later date.

Severe concussion (grade III) is likely to present with a comatose and paralysed athlete. After some minutes he or she may pass through various stages of stupor, confusion, delirium and automatic movements before regaining consciousness. Retrograde and antegrade amnesia will be present. Repeated neurological examinations should be carried out to ensure that he or she has not also got an intracranial hemorrhage or a cervicospinal injury. He or she should be carried off on a spine board or stretcher and admitted to hospital for at least 24 hours. He or she should not engage in competitions for at least a month, or participate again in a sport which is likely to cause brain injury.

SPORTS INJURIES AND DISORDERS

Contusion

Contusion is a hemorrhage into soft tissue without a break in the skin.

Muscle contusion can cause a hematoma, edema, inflammation, pain and disability. Myositis ossificans is a complication. Treatment involves the use of ice, compression, non-steroidal anti-inflammatory drugs and graduated muscle stretching exercises.

Coracoid process stress fracture

Stress fracture of the coracoid process of the scapula can occur in baseball pitchers. At the time of the fracture the pitcher is likely to complain of an acute pain in the shoulder on pitching. This can be followed by chronic pain or discomfort.

Corns and calluses

Corns and calluses can develop on the hands of rowers or on the feet of runners and football players who wear badly-fitting shoes or boots.

Costochondral separation

Costochondral separation can occur as a result of a direct blow to the chest. Clinical features are a sharp localized pain followed by an intermittent stabbing pain and sometimes a visible and palpable lump. The cartilage can click back into place and out again several times over a few days before healing takes place. Occasionally there is non-union and the dislocation is chronic. Treatment involves the use of ice and analgesics. For persistent pain a local anesthetic can be injected under strict aseptic conditions. Permanent dislocation may require the excision of a segment of cartilage.

Cotton's test

Cotton's test assesses the mediolateral movement of the talus in the ankle joint in tibiofibular syndesmosis injuries. One hand stabilizes the distal lower leg while the thumb and forefinger of the other hand grasp the foot at the talus. By the application of mediolateral force instability and crepitus are assessed. Movement of over 3 mm in this plane is an indication of probable diastasis.

Cubital tunnel syndrome

Cubital tunnel syndrome is due to compression of the ulnar nerve at the elbow. It can occur as an overuse condition in throwers, tennis players, badminton players and weight-lifters. The compression can be due to either muscular, aponeurotic or bony abnormalities at the elbow. Clinical features are pain down the medial side of the forearm, paresthesiae and eventually anesthesia of the ulnar one and a half digits, a feeling of clumsiness in the hand and wasting of the muscles of the hand supplied by the ulnar nerve. Treatment can be non-operative with rest, elbow pads and ice, or operative if these measures fail.

Cyclist's pain

Cyclist's can develop back pain, which is often relieved by altering the saddle height, or knee pain if they ride on a bicycle with the saddle too low.

Cyclist purpuric lesions

Purpuric spots can develop in the skin of a cyclist's forearms if he or she rests their forearms on the handlebars when riding over wet ground.

D

Dead arm syndrome

Other name Javelin thrower's shoulder

Dead arm syndrome is an injury of the shoulder that can occur in sports which involve throwing an object such as a javelin. It occurs during the acceleration phase of throwing and is due to a momentary subluxation of the glenohumeral joint associated with compression of the brachial plexus. The patient complains of the arm suddenly becoming useless and dropping down by his or her side; he or she may also complain of pins and needles in it. Recovery takes place in a few seconds or minutes. Treatment is directed towards stabilizing the joint.

Dead leg

Dead leg is the result of a kick or other blow on a leg muscle causing an acute hemorrhage into the muscle. The patient feels severe pain and falls to the ground with muscle spasm. A painful lump may persist at the spot for several weeks. Treatment involves rest, ice, compression and elevation of the limb.

Decompression sickness

Decompression sickness can occur in scuba divers. The following clinical features can occur singly or in combination.

(a) *Pain*: a dull pain usually affects the large joints and can initially flit from one joint to another but later becomes more severe and localized; there may be limitation of movement and girdle pain.

(b) *Neurological symptoms*: any dysfunction of the central and peripheral nervous systems can occur; this may include disturbances of behavior, mood, speech, intelligence, consciousness, motor and sensory function, cerebellar functions and loss of sphincter control (especially of the bladder).

(c) *Audiovestibular disturbances*: nausea, vomiting, nystagmus, tinnitus, vertigo and deafness.

(d) *Pulmonary symptoms*: cough, dyspnea, cyanosis, chest pain, hemoptysis and cardiopulmonary collapse.

(e) *Skin features*: erythematous rash, itching and 'suit squeeze' (dark reticulate marks on the skin due to compression of creases of skin by the diving suit).

(f) *Other features* can be fatigue, headache, malaise, loss of appetite, lymphedema and lymphadenopathy.

Immediate treatment involves the administration of 100% oxygen from a demand system, oral fluid to fully conscious patients with a good airway or an intravenous infusion of crystalloid solution. The bladder may have to be catherized.

See also Scuba diver's decompression sickness

Deep peroneal nerve entrapment
See Anterior tarsal syndrome

Deep-water blackout

Deep-water blackout is a sudden loss of consciousness in divers on air below about 70 m. Physical exercises can precipitate this condition. The cause is a combination of increased oxygen partial pressure, increased carbon dioxide and nitrogen bubbling followed by necrosis. Recovery is likely to be rapid if the swimmer maintains his or her air supply.

Deltoid ligament injury

Injury of the deltoid ligament in the ankle can be either a sprain or a complete rupture which usually occurs on the lateral side and can be associated with a Maisonneuve fracture. Clinical features are pain, tenderness, swelling, bruising and an inability to bear weight on the leg or to walk. Treatment of a sprain involves rest and non-steroid anti-inflammatory drugs; treatment of a rupture may be conservative or surgical.

Dementia pugilistica
See Punch-drunk syndrome

Dental injuries

Dental injuries are due to direct blows and can be either crown fractures, root fractures, dentoalveolar fractures or avulsion of teeth. They can be associated with facial injuries, soft tissue lacerations, fractures of facial bones and brain injury. Fragments of broken teeth may be inhaled or embedded in a lip. The prognosis is good with immediate treatment. An avulsed permanent tooth should be replaced immediately.

de Quervain's syndrome

de Quervain's syndrome is tenosynovitis of the abductor pollicis longus and extensor pollicis brevis and can be due to to repetitive deviation movements. Clinical features are pain, swelling and tenderness at the styloid process of the radius. Ulnar deviation of the wrist with the thumb fully adducted causes severe pain (Finkelstein's test). Treatment involves rest from sporting activities, splinting and non-steroidal anti-inflammatory drugs. If these fail, surgery is required to release the first dorsal compartment.

See also Finkelstein's test

Destot's sign

Destot's sign is a large superficial hematoma beneath the inguinal ligament or in the scrotum due to a fracture of the pelvis.

Digital artery thrombosis

Thrombosis of the digital arteries can occur in the catching hand of baseball and handball players, with the fingers becoming white and numb. Ulceration and gangrene can be complications.

Digital collateral ligament injuries

Collateral ligament injuries of the fingers are likely in footballers, soccer players, baseball players and basketball players. The injury can be either a partial or a complete rupture of the digital collateral ligament. Clinical features are pain, swelling and loss of movement. With a partial injury a player may carry on playing and suffer further injury, perhaps converting a partial rupture into a complete one. Treatment of a partial rupture involves taping or immobilization. A complete rupture can be treated by immobilization or surgery.

Disability rating scale

Disability rating scale is an assessment of a patient's abilities after a brain injury such as concussion. The different categories evaluated are assessed using the methods shown in Table 1 and assigned a rating score. The sum of the scores indicates the level of disability (Table 2).

Table 1 The methods used to assess each category evaluated by the disability rating score which evaluates a patient's abilities after a brain injury

Category	Method of assessment
Arousability	eye opening
Awareness and responsibility	commuication ability motor response
Cognitive ability for self-care and activities	feeding, toileting, grooming
Dependence on others	degree of dependence
Psychosocial adaptability	employability

Table 2 How the sum of the scores (total score) assigned to the categories shown in Table 1 determines the level of a patient's disabilities following a brain injury

Total score	Level of disability
0	none
1	mild
2–3	partial
4–6	moderate
7–11	moderately severe
12–16	severe
17–21	extremely severe
22–24	vegetative state
25–29	extreme vegetative state

Distal phalangeal fracture

Fracture of a distal phalanx in American football and rugby occurs as a tuft or shaft fracture due to the bone being crushed. In basketball and softball the bone is subjected to an axial load and the fracture may involve the joint. Clinical features are pain, swelling and bruising under the nail. Treatment of a simple fracture involves splinting from the interphalangeal joint to the finger tip for about 6 weeks or until he or she is free from pain, but a displaced or comminuted fracture requires reduction and pinning under a digital block.

Distal posterior interosseous nerve syndrome

Distal posterior interosseous nerve syndrome describes a pain in the wrist which is thought to be due to compression or irritation of the terminal sensory division of the posterior interosseous nerve as it passes over the distal end of the radius and enters the dorsal wrist capsule. The pain can be produced by forceful wrist extension and deep palpation of the dorsum of the wrist when it is in flexion.

See also Posterior interosseous syndrome

Distal radial fracture

Distal radial fracture with the closed rupture of the extensor indicis tendon can occur in gymnasts who grip so tightly on the bar that rotation is prevented.

Diving injuries

Injuries due to diving into shallow swimming pools, rivers, lakes and ponds can be scalp lacerations, closed head injuries, cervico-spinal injuries, as well as fractures of the ribs, thoracic vertebrae, pelvis and other bones, near-drowning and multiple organ failure syndrome. It is commonly associated with a high blood alcohol level.

Dorsal root ganglion syndrome

Dorsal root ganglion syndrome is characterized by severe pain in the arm following a cervical hyperflexion or hyperextension injury. The pain is made worse by extension or flexion of the head. There is usually no sensory loss. It is thought to be due to contusion and hemorrhage into and around the dorsal root ganglia in the neck.

Drop finger
See Mallet finger

E

Ear drum injury

Ear drum injury is due to a direct blow to the head which produces a tear of the drum. Clinical features are bleeding from the external auditory meatus, pain and dizziness. Healing usually takes place in 6 weeks and during that time the player should not engage in any sport in which he or she might receive another blow to the head.

Earle's sign

Earle's sign is a large hematoma or bony prominence felt on rectal examination which is due to, and a sign of, a pelvic fracture.

See also Pelvic bone fractures

Effort thrombosis

Other names Axillary vein thrombosis, Paget–von Schrötter syndrome, subclavian vein thrombosis

Effort thrombosis can occur in baseball, football and handball players, in swimmers and in contact sports players. Excessive stretching of the arm causes thromboses of the subclavian and axillary veins. It is more common in men than women and most common in the fourth decade of life. Clinical features are swelling and cyanosis of the arm, a feeling of heaviness, discomfort or coolness in the arm and a visible enlargement of collateral veins over the shoulder. The thrombosis may be palpable in the axilla or medial aspect of the arm. Complications are gangrene of the arm and pulmonary embolism. Treatment involves rest from sporting activities, a sling and fibrinolytic therapy. Surgery may be necessary.

Effort thrombosis can occur in the leg veins of a runner and cause pain in the calf.

Elbow dislocation

Dislocation of the elbow is usually due to a fall on an outstretched hand and can occur in any contact sport. Associated conditions are fracture of the head of the radius, of the olecranon and coracoid process of the ulna, of the medial and lateral epicondyles of the humerus, and of the capitellum; other complications are median nerve entrapment and brachial artery injury. The dislocation, which is obvious, can be followed by muscle spasm and swelling. Treatment of an uncomplicated dislocation involves reduction as soon as possible, if necessary under an anesthetic. The growth of ectopic bone can be a complication of a fracture/dislocation.

Elbow flexion contracture

Elbow flexion contracture can occur in baseball pitchers and throwers either suddenly or after years of these sporting activities. It can also be due to hyperextension of the joint during base sliding in baseball or when colliding with another player in any sport. A painful acute contracture should be treated with rest from sport until free from pain, non-steroidal anti-inflammatory drugs and passive stretching exercise.

Ely's test

Ely's test is a assessment of rectus femoris contraction. If it is positive the patient cannot completely flex the knee with the hip fully extended.

Enthesopathy

Enthesopathy is a strain of muscle, ligament or tendon attachments. It can occur as tibialis anterior strain in young footballers, extensor strain in tennis and rackets players, elbow spondylitis in golf, tennis and rackets players, and shin pain in runners. Treatment involves rest from the sport, correction of any cause, local corticoid injection and physiotherapy.

Epidural hematoma

Epidural hematoma is due to a tear of the middle meningeal artery in its bony canal in the skull or, less frequently, of some other meningeal artery, and the formation of a large clot. Clinical features are varied. The patient may either (a) become unconscious and remain unconscious; (b) become unconscious, have a period of consciousness and then become unconscious again; or (c) may not develop consciousness until later. He or she should be admitted to hospital and have a CT scan to identify the site of the lesion.

Erythrasma

Erythrasma is characterized by dull reddish-brown plaques in intertriginous areas (i.e. the axillae and groins) due to infection by *Corynebacterium minutissimum*. Treatment involves washing with soap and water and the application of an antibiotic solution.

Excessive lateral hypercompression syndrome

See Patellofemoral pain syndrome

Exertional headache

Other name Cephalalgia

Exertional headache is a headache occurring during resistance training. It is usually a benign condition which subsides with rest from the training, but the athlete should be medically examined in case it is due to a serious intracranial condition (e.g. an aneurysm).

Extensor digitorum communis tendonitis

Extensor digitorum communis tendonitis is a non-infective, painful inflammation of the tendons attributed to their compression by over-tight laces. Treatment is by rest, warm soaks, analgesics and non-steroidal anti-inflammatory drugs.

External oblique muscle strain

External oblique muscle strain is a detachment, partial or complete, of fibres of the muscle from their attachment to the iliac crest. It is most likely to occur in players of American football and ice hockey. The patient complains of very severe pain and tenderness in the iliac crest and of difficulty in straightening the trunk. Immediate treatment involves rest, ice, compression, taping and abdominal binding. Taping should be continued when the patient returns to his or her sport and protective padding may be necessary. Surgical repair is sometimes needed.

F

Fabella syndrome

The fabella is a sesamoid bone which in 12% of the normal population is present in the tendinous portion of the lateral head of gastrocnemius; it can be bilateral. Its anterior surface articulates with the posterior surface of the lateral femoral condyle. The syndrome, which can occur in adolescence or adult life, is due to roughening of the articular surface, tendonitis, synovial irritation or fracture of the fabella. It is characterized by pain in the posterolateral aspect of the knee and localized tenderness. Diagnosis can usually be made by X-ray, but in adolescence the fabella may not be ossified. Treatment involves rest, nonsteroidal anti-inflammatory drugs and the injection of a corticosteroid and a local anesthetic. Surgical removal may be necessary.

Facial laceration

Facial laceration can occur in boxing, wrestling, cricket and other sports. It is most common in the lips and eyebrow region. Treatment involves compression and dressing, as well as irrigation and suturing for a deep laceration.

Fat embolus

Fat embolus is a complication of a long bone fracture. Clinical features are petechiae, anemia, pyrexia, rapid respiration, thrombocytopenia, a Pa_{O_2} less than 60 mmHg on air, the need for ventilatory support and X-rays showing diffuse infiltration of the lungs.

Femoral epiphysial fracture

Femoral epiphysial fracture can occur in adolescent basketball and volleyball players before full skeletal maturity has been achieved. It can be due to deceleration after a run or hyper-extension of the knee when landing from a jump. Clinical features are severe pain, swelling and inability to stand on the leg. Treatment involves closed reduction and a cast. A severe fracture may require surgery.

Femoral head dislocation

Femoral head dislocation is generally in a posterior direction. The athlete is in extreme pain and immobilized, with the leg held in flexion, internal rotation and adduction. In the rarer anterior dislocation it is held in flexion, external rotation and abduction, and the head of the femur may be palpable. No attempt at reduction should be made on the spot and the patient is transported to hospital for reduction of the dislocation.

Femoral neck fracture

Fracture of the femur neck is uncommon in young athletes, because of the great force necessary to produce it, and occurs more frequently in older sportswomen with osteoporotic bone. Clinical features are sudden severe pain, inability to bear weight on the leg, and shortening and external rotation of the leg. The fracture may be transepiphyseal (with or without dislocation), transcervical, cervicotrochanteric or intertrochanteric. Complications are injury to the growth plate causing a varus deformity of the femoral neck and head, and loss of vascularity in the femoral head with avascular necrosis of it. Treatment is by immobilization in a spica cast or internal fixation with a pin.

Stress fracture of the femoral neck can occur in runners and other athletes. Risk factors are coxa vara, bad footwear and poor running surfaces. Clinical features are either pain in the groin, anterior thigh or knee, or an aching sensation which disappears with cessation of activity, limitation of hip movement (especially internal rotation) and pain produced by percussion or compression of the greater trochanter. An X-ray may not show anything abnormal for 2–4 weeks. Compression fracture is more common in young athletes, while a transverse fracture usually occurs in older athletes and is likely to displace if placed under further stress. Treatment involves bed rest until the patient is pain-free, then by non-weight-bearing ambulation on crutches, with return to full activity when X-rays show a healed fracture. Displacement requires immediate reduction and internal fixation.

Femoral nerve tension test

See Reverse straight-leg raising test

Femoral shaft stress fracture

Femoral shaft stress fracture occurs in runners and joggers. Risk factors are unsuitable running shoes, an increase in the intensity and duration of the activity, change in running surface and osteopenia (which is common in amenorrheal or oligomenorrheal women athletes). The fracture can occur anywhere along the shaft, but is usually at the junction of the proximal and middle third; it can be bilateral. The patient usually complains of slight pain which is relieved by rest and made worse by running; he/she may also complain of a severe sudden pain and rarely of little pain before displacement of the fracture occurs. Clinical features are local tenderness, swelling at the site, limitation of movement and an increase in pain with axial loading or forced rotation. Treatment involves the use of crutches to prevent weight-bearing, with progression to full weight-bearing in 2–4 weeks, and by non-weight-bearing activities such as swimming and cycling. Running can usually be resumed in 8–16 weeks.

Femoral subtrochanteric stress fracture

Subtrochanteric stress fracture of the femur is a rare condition which can present with progressive pain in the hip or upper thigh. An X-ray may not reveal the lesion, for which a bone scan is necessary. Treatment involves using crutches with partial weight-bearing until free from pain.

Femoral upper epiphysis slip

Femoral upper epiphysis slip can occur as an acute or chronic condition in adolescents who have not attained full skeletal maturity. Clinical features of an acute slip are severe pain in the hip, inability to bear weight on the leg and an external rotation hip contracture.

Fibular and tibial stress fracture

Stress fracture of the fibula and tibia can occur in runners and jumpers. They are more common in the tibia than in the fibula and, like other stress fractures, they are more common in women than men. Clinical features are pain, tenderness and, occasionally, periosteal thickening and callus formation. Treatment involves rest from sporting activities until free from pain and then a gradual return, with full return likely in 3–4 months.

Fifth metatarsal stress fracture

Other name Jones' fracture

Stress fracture of the fifth metatarsal can occur just distal to its base in runners, jumpers and players of American football and volleyball. It presents with pain and tenderness. Treatment involves rest from activities that aggravate the injury and by immobilization for 6–8 weeks. Complications are delayed union and non-union.

Finkelstein's test

Finkelstein's test is a test for de Quervain's syndrome. In this condition ulnar deviation of the wrist with the thumb fully adducted causes severe pain.

See also de Quervain's syndrome

Flexor digitorum profundus avulsion

Flexor digitorum profundus avulsion can occur in players of American football and basketball; usually in the ring finger. A bony fragment may be avulsed. Clinical features are pain, swelling, tenderness and an inability to flex the terminal interphalangeal joint. Treatment is surgical.

Flexor hallucis longus laceration

Laceration of the flexor hallucis longus has occurred in runners running barefoot and treading on a piece of glass or other sharp object.

Flexor–pronator tendonitis

Flexor–pronator tendonitis is a strain of the flexors of the wrist and pronators of the forearm, which can occur in baseball pitchers who have a poor throwing technique. Clinical features are discomfort in the muscles and tenderness. Treatment involves rest from throwing and learning the correct action.

Fracture union, non-union, malunion

Fracture union is a complex process which restores the full integrity of part of the skeleton with bone that is indistinguishable from the original material. Remodelling is usually so perfect that all evidence of a fracture can disappear.

A fracture that has not united by 4 months is considered to have delayed union. Non-union is defined as a failure to unite by 6 months, with radiological evidence that it is going to be permanent if there is no intervention. Radiological categories are either (a) atrophic, with narrow round osteoporotic bone; or (b) hypertrophic, with excessive bone formation. Fractures with a high risk of delayed union or malunion are fractures into a joint and high-energy fractures with soft tissue stripping. Tibial, scaphoid, femoral neck and intracapsular femoral fractures are the ones particularly likely to have delayed union or non-union. Conditions associated with delayed union and non-union are osteogenesis imperfecta, rickets, scurvy, diabetes mellitus, rheumatoid arthritis, Osgood–Schlatter disease (tibial tuberosity fracture), and human immunodeficiency virus (HIV) infection. Delayed union and non-union are uncommon in children.

Malunion is a union with an anatomical abnormality that affects the function of all, or a part of, the patient.

Freiberg's disease

Freiberg's disease is an avascular necrosis of a metatarsal head, usually the second or third phalanx. It is a result of jumping or sprinting by young athletes and occurs most frequently in those with Morton's foot (short first toe, long second toe). Clinical features are pain, swelling and stiffness in the metatarsophalangeal joint. Fragmentation of the bone can occur. Treatment involves rest from sport, wearing a metatarsal relief pad and, sometimes, wearing a short walking cast. Surgery is necessary to remove any fragment.

Frostbite

Frostbite can develop when the climatic temperature falls below 0°C. It can be superficial, in which there is only a little loss of tissue, or deep, in which there is serious tissue loss. Clinical features of superficial frostbite are white, bluish or mottled color of the affected part, loss of sensation and mobility of the skin over bony points. In deep frostbite the affected part is very hard and the skin over bony points may be immobile. Thawing can cause erythema, painful swelling and blister formation in hours or days, which is followed by the formation of a dry eschar and mummification. In superficial frostbite new epithelium forms. In deep frostbite dead tissue is demarcated from healthy tissue and autoamputation can occur. Treatment is by rapid rewarming in water at 40°–42°C for up to 30 minutes; the pain is severe and analgesic drugs may be necessary. This is followed by open exposure, with digits separated by lambswool, using cradle to keep bedclothes off the injured part and hydrotherapy. Rewarming should not be attempted in the field and exposure to an open fire can cause a thermal burn. Surgical amputation may be performed after demarcation of the dead area is established. Frostbite can be prevented by wearing proper clothing and boots.

Complications can be infection causing wet gangrene, atrophy of digit fat pads and premature closure of epiphyses in children with arrest of growth in the frostbitten part. Corneal injuries may be cold-induced lesions.

See also Hypothermia

Frostnip

Frostnip is due to exposure of the skin to the cold and is less severe than frostbite. The skin is insensitive, painful and white, but is pliable. Treatment involves warming the affected the part under clothing or if possible in the armpit, whereupon it returns to normal in a few minutes.

G

Gaenslen's test

Gaenslen's test confirms the presence of a sacroiliac strain. With the patient lying supine, the examiner hyperflexes the hip on the unaffected side in order to lock the pelvis and then hyperextends the hip on the affected side. The production of pain is a positive response.

Gastrocnemius tear

See Tennis leg

Gastrocnemius tendonitis

Gastrocnemius tendonitis can occur as an overuse injury in long-distance runners. Clinical features are pain in the muscle and down the leg, tenderness over the head of gastrocnemius and pain when fully resisting knee flexion while the patient is lying prone. Treatment involves rest, ice, non-steroidal anti-inflammatory drugs and the injection of a local anesthetic and a corticosteroid.

Gerber's test

Gerber's test evaluates the function of the subscapularis muscle. The patient places the arm in internal rotation with the dorsum of the hand on the back pocket of his or her trousers. If he or she is unable to internally rotate the arm any further and to lift the hand off the pocket, then the subscapularis is probably ruptured and incompetent.

Glasgow coma scale (modified)

The Glasgow coma scale aims to measure the depth of a coma. This involves assessing a set of features and then allocating the patient the score which has been set for that particular response by the patient. As can be seen in Table 3, each feature is scored separately, with the patient attaining a minimum of 3 and maximum of 15 points. The total is a quantitative index of the level of cerebral function.

Table 3 The score allocated to each feature assessed in the Glasgow coma scale. This provides a quantitative index of cerebral function

Feature assessed	Score allocated
Eyes open:	
spontaneously	4
to speech	3
to pain	2
none	1
Eyes closed due to swelling	C*
Best verbal response:	
orientated	5
confused	4
inappropriate words	3
incomprehensible sounds	2
none	1
Endotracheal tube *in situ* or tracheostomy	T*
Best motor response:	
obeys command	6
localizes pain	5
flexion withdrawal	4
decerebrate flexion	3
decerebrate extension	2
none	1

* In these cases the patient is unable to be assessed on the feature. C = eyes closed, T = endotracheal tube/tracheostomy

Glasgow coma scale for children

Modified version of the Glasgow coma scale which aims to measure the depth of a coma in young children. In a similar manner to the scale for adults, this involves assessing a set of features and then allocating the patient the score which has been set for that particular response by the patient. As can be seen in Table 4, each feature is scored separately, with the patient attaining a minimum of 3 and a maximum of 15 points. While the total is a quantitative index of the level of cerebral function, the normal developmental milestones have to be taken into account. Thus, the interpretation of the total scores has to take into consideration the maximum score that can be attained by children under 5 years (see Table 5).

Table 4 The score allocated to each feature assessed in the Glasgow coma scale for children. This provides a quantitative index of cerebral function

Feature assessed	Score allocated
Eyes open:	
spontaneously	4
to speech	3
to pain	2
none	1
Eyes closed due to swelling	C*
Best verbal response:	
orientated	5
words	4
vocal sounds	2
none	1
Endotracheal tube *in situ* or tracheostomy	T*
Best motor response:	
obeys command	6
localizes pain	5
flexion withdrawal	4
flexion extension	3
decerebrate extension	2
none	1

*In these cases the patient is unable to be assessed on the feature. C = eyes closed, T = endotracheal tube/tracheostomy

Table 5 The maximum score that can be attained by children of different ages from the Glasgow coma scale for children. The normal developmental milestones have to be taken into consideration if an appropriate assessment of cerebral function is to be made

Age (in months)	Maximum score possible
0–6	9
6–12	11
12–24	12
24–60	13
> 60	15

Glasgow outcome scale

The Glasgow outcome scale is an assessment of survival, social integration and daily living abilities after a brain injury. Table 6 shows how the scores allocated in the five-point system are used to predict the outcome for the patient.

Table 6 The predicted outcome of patients from scores allocated according to the five-point Glasgow outcome scale. This provides an indication of the patient's abilities after a brain injury

Score allocated	Predicted outcome
1	death due to brain injury usually follows within 48 hours
2	persistent vegetative state
3	severe disability; the patient will be concious but disabled and dependent on others for daily living
4	partial recovery, with work at a simpler level
5	good recovery, with a normal life style and return to work; minor neurophysical/neurobehavioral sequelae may be present

Glenohumeral subluxation and dislocation

See Shoulder joint subluxation and dislocation

Glenoid labrum tear

Glenoid labrum tear can occur in sports which involve throwing an object such as the javelin. Recurrent subluxation of the shoulder is an associated condition. Clinical features are painful clicks, locking of the shoulder and, sometimes, tenderness on deep palpation. The diagnosis can be confirmed by arthrotomography or magnetic resonance imaging. A loose portion of the labrum may be removed by arthroscopic resection.

Golfer's elbow

Golfer's elbow is a medial epicondylitis of the humerus and is characterized by pain and tenderness at the site. Treatment involves rest, ice and oral non-steroidal anti-inflammatory drugs.

See also Medial epicondylitis, Tenoperiostitis

Groin disruption syndrome

Groin disruption syndrome is characterized by a torn external oblique aponeurosis, a torn conjoint tendon and dehiscence between the conjoint tendon and the inguinal ligament. The patient complains of pain in the inguinal, adductor or perianal region. The pain is made worse by sudden changes of movement and prevents kicking a ball.

H

Haglund's syndrome
See Retrocalcaneal bursitis

Hamate fractures

Hamate fractures can occur on the body or the hook of the bone. It can be due to a blow on the hypothenar eminence from a baseball bat, golf club, hockey stick or tennis racket. Clinical features are weak grip, wrist pain and tenderness over the fracture. Treatment of a non-displaced fracture of the body involves immobilization for 4–6 weeks. A displaced fracture of the body is treated surgically. Complications of a hook fracture can be displacement of the fractured piece, tendonitis, ulnar nerve impingement and rupture of the flexor tendon of the little finger due to chronic inflammation. The fracture is difficult to see radiographically. Non-union is common and, if the condition does not respond to conservative treatment involving rest and a short-arm cast, surgical removal of the hook may be necessary.

Hammer finger
See Mallet finger

Hamstring muscle strain and rupture

Hamstring muscle strain is a common injury. Risk factors are an inadequate warm up, poor technique and endurance, imbalance of muscle strength (hamstring-to-quadriceps and hamstring-to-hamstring) and inequality of leg length. The strain occurs at musculotendinous junctions, which in the hamstrings run almost the complete length. The athlete complains of a sudden pain in the back of the thigh, may feel a tearing sensation and may hear a 'pop'. Clinical examination reveals localized tenderness over the strain, bruising and sometimes a palpable mass or a gap if the

injury is severe. Treatment involves rest, ice, compression, elevation of the limb and non-steroidal anti-inflammatory drugs,
followed by protective exercises, pre- and post-exercise passive
stretching, and a gradual return to full activity.

Heat rash
See Prickly heat

Heat syndromes

Heat syndromes are, in order of severity: heat cramp, heat
syncope, heat collapse, heat exhaustion and heat stroke. An
athlete can pass from one into another. They are most likely to
occur on a hot day with high solar radiation, a high relative
humidity and little or no wind, in athletes who are not heat-
acclimatized and inadequately hydrated.

Heat cramps are painful spasms of large muscle groups, usually
the gastrocnemius and soleus and the hamstrings and extensors
of the legs. They are due to dehydration and low serum sodium
and chloride. Prevention is by adequate hydration before exercise. As an athlete may refuse to drink large amounts of a salty
solution, an intravenous injection of 1–1.5 l of normal saline
solution may have to be given.

Heat syncope is due to an athlete standing in the sun after an
event. It is a transient fainting episode due to venous pooling and
decreased cardiac output and stroke volume. The core body
temperature is normal. Treatment involves lying down in the
shade. Oral hydration is needed if the athlete is dehydrated.

Heat collapse can occur both in athletes and in spectators who
have been standing for a long time and is characterized by loss
of consciousness due to an inadequate cerebral blood flow. Treatment involves lying down, elevation of the legs, tepid sponging
and fluids by mouth when consciousness has been regained.

Heat exhaustion is a severe form of heat intolerance. Clinical
features are fatigue, thirst, confusion, nausea and vomiting. It
may be the result of either water or salt depletion. The sodium
depletion may be due to a deficiency of dietary sodium chloride
or to high sodium chloride loss in sweating. Treatment involves
giving oral fluid for water depletion and sodium chloride solution by intravenous injection for sodium chloride deficiency.

Heat stroke is an extremely serious condition and can be fatal.
Early symptoms are excessive sweating, headache, nausea,
muscle aching and disturbance of consciousness. It can present
very rapidly, with a high temperature (core temperature of over

41°C), clouding of consciouness, delirium (sometimes with hallucinations), muscular twitching, seizures and loss of control of the sphincters. Other features can be tachycardia, cardiac arrhythmias, hypotension, myoglobinuria and hepatic impairment. A very high core temperature can cause irreversible damage to the brain, liver, kidneys and adrenal glands. Death is most likely to be due to circulatory failure. Immediate treatment involves removal to a cool place, tepid sponging and fanning. Cooling by ice, cold sponging and fanning with cold air are forbidden as they increase the heat by causing vasoconstriction. If there is no immediate improvement, the patient should be hospitalized.

Heel pain

Other name Calcaneodynia

Heel pain is a common condition in runners and long-distance walkers. They complain of either pain of acute onset following a twist of the ankle or of a pain slowly developing on the medial side of the bottom of the heel. The pain is bad on getting up in the morning, can decrease with activity, and then increase with further activity. If the pain is severe the patient is unable to put any weight on the heel and stands on the front of his or her foot. There may be tenderness over the medial tuberosity of the calcaneus. Various views to its cause are held. It has been attributed to bony spurs of the calcaneus, inflammation, plantar fascia pull, irritation of the medial calcaneal nerve, entrapment of the motor nerve to abductor digiti quinti (minimi), and herniation and compression of fat nodules. Sarcoidosis is a risk factor. Various treatments are suggested. If bony spurs are present they can be removed. Other treatments are immobilization, nonsteroidal anti-inflammatory drugs, plantar fasciotomy and surgical treatment of nerves that might be responsible.

Heel-spur syndrome

Other name Plantar fasciitis

Heel-spur syndrome is a common cause of heel pain in runners. Chronic traction on the plantar aponeurosis at its insertion into the calcaneus produces an inflammatory reaction and sometimes a bony spur. Pain starts at the beginning of running and may diminish during it, only to recur afterwards. The heel may also be painful during the patient's first steps in the morning. Tenderness does occur in the medial half of the plantar fascia distal to its insertion into calcaneus and at the insertion of abductor hallucis into calcaneus; this is due to overuse of the muscle while trying to walk with the foot inverted.

Hematuria

Hematuria can occur after any severe sporting activity and should resolve spontaneously without causing any trouble. After an event marathon runners usually have temporary microscopic hematuria (the presence of more than two red cells per high-power field in a centrifuged specimen of urine; this is in the absence of menstrual blood in women).

Hepatitis B infection

Hepatitis B infection in athletes is usually acquired by either using infected towels, brushes, and soaps in common washrooms or by person-to-person contact in steam baths. Barefoot runners have been infected by stepping on thorns infected by a previous barefoot runner.

Herpes gladiatorum

Herpes gladiatorum is a herpes simplex infection of the skin acquired in wrestling with an infected wrestler, or from tackling an infected rugby or football player. Clinical features are grouped vesicles on erythematous bases. An infected athlete should not take part in any contact sport.

High altitude disorders

Other names Acute mountain sickness, mountaineering disorders

High altitudes are those over 1500 m (5000 feet). At altitudes above 2500 m the low barometric pressure produces a lower inspired partial pressure of oxygen, impairment of oxygen transport, a reduction in the transfer of oxygen across the alveolar–capillary membrane and a reduction in the binding of oxygen to hemoglobin. High altitude disorders occur in mountain climbers, balloonists, gliders, hang-gliders, parachutists, aviators, skiers and marathon runners. Preventive measures include gradual acclimatization by slow ascent, high-carbohydrate intake, low salt intake, adequate hydration and reduced workload at arrival. Contraindications to climbing to high altitudes are pregnancy, cardiovascular disease, pulmonary disease, hypertension and anemia. The high altitude disorders are acute mountain sickness, cerebral edema, pulmonary edema and retinal hemorrhage.

Acute mountain sickness usually occurs within 24–72 hours from the start of the climb. It is characterized by fatigue, shortness of breath, headache, nausea, vomiting, Cheyne–Stokes respiration, generalized edema and insomnia. It can be prevented and treated with acetazolamide and is usually a mild and self-limited disease lasting for 24–48 hours. If it persists beyond that time, the climber should descend immediately. If he or she does not, a severe illness can develop with retinal hemorrhage, blurring of vision and temporary blindness.

Cerebral edema can occur at over 3500 m (11 000 feet) and develops over 2–3 days. Fluid extravasates from the vascular to the extravascular space, causing tissue edema and increased intracranial pressure. Clinical features are severe headache, confusion, hallucinations and hypercoagulability. Fits, hemiparesis, stupor and coma can develop with a risk of permanent neurological complications or death. Treatment involves descent and admission to hospital.

Pulmonary edema is characterized by shortness of breath, cough, cyanosis, increased respiratory rate, increased heart rate, pulmonary hypertension and frothy sputum. It occurs at over 2400 m (8000 feet) after 1–4 days at that height in fit, acclimatized climbers and skiers, and is fatal in 10% of cases. Treatment involves descent and admission to hospital.

Retinal hemorrhage can be benign and symptomless (unless it involves the macula, causing scotoma or a blind spot) and resolves spontaneously within 1–2 weeks after descent.

Hill–Sachs lesion

Hill–Sachs lesion is an impacted or compression fracture of the head of the humerus associated with anterior dislocation of the head. It is due to compression or recoil impaction of the head against the rim of the glenoid fossa at the moment of dislocation.

Hip contusion

Hip contusion is due to a direct blow, commonly over one of the bony prominences. Hemorrhage can occur and be persistent. Treatment involves applying pressure to stop the hemorrhage, ice and rest.

Hip dislocation

Hip dislocation occurs posteriorly in 85–92% and anteriorly in 8–15%. The patient is immediately disabled and in acute pain. In posterior dislocation the leg is held in flexion, adduction and internal rotation. In anterior dislocation it is held in flexion, abduction and external rotation; the head of the femur may be palpable. Treatment is by immobilization and removal to an appropriate treatment center for X-ray and reduction. Any intra-articular body found by X-ray should be removed arthroscopically if possible. After reduction light skin traction is applied for 48 hours. Weight-bearing is allowed progressively, with full weight-bearing in 3–4 weeks. Recurrent instability can be a complication.

Hip pointer

Hip pointer is a contusion of the iliac crest, which is characterized by pain, tenderness and swelling due to a blow or a fall on the side. Treatment involves using ice, compression and non-steroidal anti-inflammatory drugs; aspiration and injection of a local anesthetic may be necessary.

'Horse-kiss'

'Horse-kiss' is a black-and-blue spot or hematoma on the outside of the thigh due to a forceful push with a knee in soccer. An effusion (which may be bloody) under the skin can rapidly become adherent to the underlying fascia. A greater effusion of blood can cause a hematoma. Treatment involves using ice, compression and after 24 hours exercise therapy (going up and down stairs, crouching and climbing onto a chair) even if it hurts.

Humeral epiphyseal separation

Humeral epiphyseal separation at the shoulder joint occurs in 11–15-year-old boys who are baseball pitchers while their skeleton is immature. The boy complains of pain in the shoulder and an inability to pitch at speed. An X-ray shows epiphyseal widening and minimal displacement. Treatment is to stop pitching.

Humeral spiral fracture

A spiral fracture of the humerus can occur in arm-wrestling, baseball and throwing sports which require a powerful rotational movement of the arm. The fracture occurs most frequently in the distal third of the bone. A complication can be the injury of the radial nerve. Treatment is conservative and involves using a hanging-arm cast, followed by strengthening exercises.

Hypertension

Hypertension can begin in early adult life and is present in 5–10% of people who are 20–30 years of age and in 20–25% of people who are 40–50 years of age. A normal blood pressure (BP) is less than 135 systolic and less than 85 diastolic, while a blood pressure of 140–159/90–104 shows borderline hypertension, one of 160/105–114 moderate hypertension, and anything higher than this is severe. Anxiety can cause a transient rise of blood pressure and so repeated examinations should be made. In women, contraceptive agents can also raise the blood pressure. Hypertension may be discovered during a routine physical examination for sports participation and is an indication for detailed examination of the cardiovascular system. Mild to moderate hypertension can be treated by slimming, a reduction in sodium chloride (salt), dietary fat and alcohol intake, and ceasing to smoke or take ergogenic aids. Athletes with borderline hypertension can engage in all sports, except possibly weight-lifting because it can cause acute rises of blood pressure. Athletes with mild to moderate hypertension whose blood pressure is controlled can engage in moderate- to high-intensity sports (e.g. baseball, basketball, distance running, hockey, rugby, soccer, swimming, tennis and basketball).

Hypothenar hammer syndrome

Hypothenar hammer syndrome is due to repetitive blunt trauma to the ulnar artery in the hand and is characterized by vasospasm, ischemia, sensitivity to cold and cramp of the hypothenar muscles. A traumatic aneurysm can develop. It is usually seen in workmen who use a hand as a hammer or handle vibrating tools, but it can occur in karate performers and volleyball players.

Hypothermia

Hypothermia can be an acute condition due to falling into icy water (usually less than 10°C) or a chronic condition in hill walkers and climbers lost in cold weather. It occurs when the core temperature falls below 35°C. Preventive measures include cancelling events in very cold weather, not going out in bad conditions and wearing the right clothing.

Mild hypothermia is a core temperature of 32–35°C, moderate hypothermia is a core temperature of 28–32°C and severe hypothermia is a core temperature below 28°C.

In *mild hypothermia* the patient is cold and pale, with vasoconstriction, shivering ataxia, uncertain hand movements, and some incoherence, disorientation and confusion. In this state a patient has been known to strip naked. The patient should be dried, covered with a blanket and, if possible, moved to a warm environment. Complete recovery will then take place.

Moderate hypothermia is a more serious condition. The patient is likely to be in a stupor or coma, with muscle rigidity, hypotension, cardiac irregularities (such as ventricular fibrillation) and dilated pupils. If heat is not added the patient is likely to die, so he or she should be covered with heating blankets, heating pads or hot-water bottles. Insertion of the trunk in a bath of warm water (40°C) can be effective, but this can be followed by rewarming shock and 'after drop'.

Severe hypothermia can also be fatal. The patient is extremely cold, comatose, with an unobtainable blood pressure, slow breathing and rigid and areflexic muscles. Treatment can involve active core rewarming, endotracheal intubation for ventilation and oxygenation, and warmed peritoneal dialysis.

In acute hypothermia due to falling overboard into cold water, the faller should adopt the HELP position (heat escape lessening position) which involves curling up and not moving.

See also Frostbite

Iliac crest apophysitis

Iliac crest apophysitis is due to multiple microscopic stress fractures causing inflammation of the iliac crest growth plate in adolescent runners before they have achieved full skeletal maturity. The runner complains of hip pain (this is how he or she will probably refer to the iliac crest) which has developed gradually over several weeks. The crest is tender and abduction is resisted. Partial avulsion of the crest can occur. Treatment involves rest for 4–6 weeks.

Iliac crest avulsion

Iliac crest avulsion can be due to spasm of the hip adductors and external oblique in adolescent players of American football before they have reached full skeletal maturity. Clinical features are pain and spasm. Treatment involves rest and positioning to relax the muscles, and then a gradual return to full activity. Non-union is a complication for which surgical excision of the un-united fragment may be necessary.

Iliac crest hematoma

Iliac crest hematoma can occur in American football and is characterized by pain, swelling, tenderness and lameness. Treatment involves ice, compression, and either steroid injection or aspiration.

Iliopectineal bursitis

Iliopectineal bursitis is an inflammation of the iliopectineal bursa between the iliopectineal ligament and the head of the femur. Clinical features are tenderness and severe pain over the anterior aspect of the thigh. To obtain relief the patient may sit in a position of hip flexion and external rotation. Treatment involves rest, non-steroidal anti-inflammatory drugs and iliopsoas tendon stretching.

Iliopsoas injury

Iliopsoas injury is a partial or complete tear at its musculotendinous junction due to a strong contraction of the muscle when the thigh is in an extended position or fixed. In adolescents, before full skeletal maturity has been reached, the lesser trochanter is likely to be avulsed. The patient complains of a sharp pain in the groin. Treatment involves rest for 4–6 weeks, protective padding and rehabilitation exercises.

Iliotibial band friction syndrome

Other name Runner's knee

Iliotibial band friction syndrome is an inflammation due to the iliotibial band rubbing against the lateral femoral condyle during running. It is an overuse syndrome which generally occurs in long-distance runners who run frequently; especially those with pronated feet or a prominent lateral epicondyle or who are bow legged. It can also be due to running in shoes with poor lateral soles. Clinical features are pain in the outer aspect of the knee and tenderness at a point over the lateral epicondyle. The pain is made worse by running up hills or walking up and down stairs. Treatment involves rest, non-steroidal anti-inflammatory drugs, shortening of the stride and not running up hills. Surgery may be necessary if these methods fail.

Impetigo

Impetigo is an infection of the skin, for which the infecting organisms are likely to be *Staphylococcus aureus*, *Streptococcus pyrogenes* and β-hemolytic streptococci. It can be transmitted from player to player in contact sports. Clinical features are a raw, red, exuding surface, pustules, and golden-yellow crusts. Some strains of the streptococci can cause glomerulonephritis and so urinalysis should be performed if they are suspected or confirmed. Treatment involves cleansing with soap or water, softening the crusts with either olive oil, sunflower oil or arachis oil, removal of the crusts using the fingers and the application of a topical antibiotic ointment (e.g. neomycin or mupirocin).

Impingement syndrome

Impingement syndrome is common in swimmers, occurring in 60% of the top swimmers (although generally not until the sixth to eighth year of their careers); it also occurs in tennis players and baseball pitchers. The syndrome can be due to inflammation following repeated impingement of the head of the humerus and of the rotator cuff muscles into the acromion. Pain is usually localized around the acromion and is most common just after the recovery phase in front crawl. Treatment involves (a) ice, non-steroidal anti-inflammatory drugs and a corticosteroid injection; (b) electrogalvanic stimulation, ultrasound and transcutaneous nerve stimulation; (c) muscle strengthening; (d) a change in swimming technique, especially to increase body roll; and (e) the use of an upper-arm band when swimming.

See also Shoulder joint instability

Infrapatellar contracture syndrome

Infrapatellar contracture syndrome is characterized by patello-femoral pain, knee stiffness and swelling and weakness of quadriceps following reconstructive knee surgery or, occasionally, a minor knee injury several weeks earlier. It is thought to be due to fibrous hyperplasia of the soft tissues in the anterior part of the knee and, in particular, of the infrapatellar pad. The condition is likely to last for weeks or months and can cause permanent disability. Treatment involves non-steroidal anti-inflammatory drugs, electrical muscle stimulation and manual mobilization of the patella. If these methods are unsuccessful surgery may be necessary.

See also Infrapatellar fat pad injury

Infrapatellar fat pad injury

Infrapatellar fat pad injury is due to an injury of the knee which produces hemorrhage and edema of the pad. Clinical features are a dull aching pain which is made worse by movement and relieved by rest, and a bulge on either side of the patellar ligament. Treatment involves rest, elevation and ice.

See also Infrapatellar contracture syndrome

Infraspinatus tendonitis

Infraspinatus tendonitis can occur in tennis players and swimmers. The site of the lesion can be at the musculotendinous junction or at the insertion of the muscle. Clinical features are pain at the back of the shoulder, tenderness at the site of the lesion, and sometimes a tender area of thickening at the musculotendinous junction. The pain is made worse by shoulder movements and radiates into the back of the arm. Treatment involves rest and the injection of a local anesthetic and a corticosteroid into the site.

Infraspinatus tendon rupture

Infraspinatus tendon rupture occurs suddenly, with pain in the posterior aspect of the shoulder. There is also disparity between active, passive and resisted movements, with the passive range of lateral rotation of the shoulder being lost. Isometric measurement shows a painless weakness in lateral rotation. Wasting of the muscle follows.

Intersection syndrome

Intersection syndrome can occur in weight-lifters and rowers. Clinical features are crepitus, pain and a 'squeaky' sensation in the radial side of the dorsal forearm at the spot where abductor pollicis longus and extensor pollicis brevis cross over the radial wrist extensors.

Intertrigo

Intertrigo is a tender inflammation of the intertriginous areas (e.g. in the axillae, submammary region and groins) and where there are overlapping folds of skin, especially in obese athletes. Candidal superinfection may be present, with pustules at the margins of affected areas. Treatment involves drying and cleaning the areas with cool compresses, using antibiotic ointment, Castellani paint or cream with antifungal or antibacterial properties, and by slimming.

Inversion stress test

Other name Talar tilt test

Inversion stress test assesses whether the calcaneofibular ligament is disrupted. It is performed by holding the heel and attempting to invert the calcaneus and talus on the tibia. If the calcaneofibular ligament is disrupted, the articular surfaces of the tibia and talus separate forming an angle called the talar tilt.

Ischial bursitis

Ischial bursitis is an inflammation of the ischial bursa with bleeding and is due to either falling on the ischial tuberosity or a severe blow. Clinical features are pain and tenderness. Treatment involves ice and non-steroidal anti-inflammatory drugs. If this is unsuccessful the bursa may need to be aspirated and injected with a corticosteroid, and as the last resort it can be excised.

Ischial tuberosity avulsion

Ischial tuberosity avulsion can occur as a result of spasm of the hamstrings in adolescent players of American football before full skeletal maturity has been reached. Clinical features are pain and spasm of the muscles. Treatment involves rest positioning to relax the hamstrings until symptom-free and a gradual return to full activity. Non-union is a complication which may require surgical excision of the un-united fragment.

Iselin's syndrome

Iselin's syndrome is tenderness, erythema and edema over the prominent base of a fifth metatarsal due to non-union of a secondary center of ossification. It is likely to occur in weight-lifters and in athletes engaged in sports which cause inversion stress on the forefoot. Treatment involves reduction in sport activities, ice and non-steroidal anti-inflammatory drugs with a short-leg walking cast if symptoms are severe.

J

Javelin thrower's shoulder
See Dead arm syndrome

Jersey finger

Other name Profundus tendon avulsion

Jersey finger is an avulsion of the flexor digitorum profundus tendon due to hyperextension of the finger (usually the ring finger) occurring when grabbing a jersey in American football or rugby. Bleeding into the flexor sheath can result in fibrosis of the sheath. Treatment is surgical.

Jogger's nipple

Jogger's nipple is a painful and sometimes fissured dermatitis of the nipple due to friction by a vest or T-shirt in joggers and runners. In women it is associated with not wearing a bra. Treatment involves applying hydrocortisone (1%). Women joggers and runners should wear a bra.

Jones' fracture
See Fifth metatarsal stress fracture

Jumper's knee

Jumper's knee is due to a small area of degeneration at the attachment of the patellar tendon to the lower pole of the patella. It can occur in athletes engaged in sports which involve jumping, such as the high jump, long jump, basketball and volleyball. It develops gradually and is not the result of a single incident. Clinical features are pain (which is reproduced by resisting active knee extension), tenderness at the lower pole of the patella and, sometimes, crepitus on passive movement of the tendon. It can be either a recurrent or a persistent disability. Treatment involves rest, ice, elevation of the leg, immobilization of the patella, injection of a corticosteroid into the tendon area (but not into the tendon) and rehabilitative exercises. Surgery is necessary if the conservative approach is unsuccessful.

K

Knee anterior cruciate ligament injury

The anterior cruciate ligament of the knee can be injured in running, jumping, skiing, American football, basketball and baseball as a result of deceleration, awkward falling from a height, twisting and cutting. It may occur as a single trauma, but it is more likely to be associated with other ligamentous or meniscal injuries of the knee. The tear can be partial or complete. There can be an avulsion fracture of the lateral tibial condyle. The patient is likely to hear or feel a 'pop'; the knee may feel as if it were hyperextended, and further activity is impossible. Hemarthrosis develops in a few hours. The patient presents with a painful swollen knee and evidence of anterior tibial subluxation. The Lachman test, pivot shift test and anterior drawer test of the knee are positive. Treatment of a young patient is surgical; an older and not very active patient can be treated conservatively with hamstring and quadriceps strengthening exercises and a derotational brace. Osteoarthritis can be a complication.

See also Anterior drawer test of the knee, Lachman's test, pivot shift test

Knee hemarthrosis

Hemarthrosis of the knee joint is usually the result of a non-contact twisting injury which has caused a tear of a cruciate ligament or, less commonly, of a meniscus. The patient may have heard a crack and presents with a swollen and painful knee. The diagnosis is confirmed by aspiration. A complication of aspiration is infection, for which the risk factors are infection of the skin at the site of aspiration, diabetes mellitus and immunosuppression.

Knee instability

Knee stability can be dynamic (provided by surrounding muscles, especially quadriceps femoris) or static (provided by ligaments). Dynamic instability is due to weakness in the inhibition of the muscles, especially vastus medialis, from any cause. Static instability can be due to injury or weakness of the capsular ligaments with loss of proprioception from them. Other causes can be a torn meniscus (especially a tear of the posterior horn of the medial mensicus), a loose foreign body in the knee, arthritis of the knee and chondromalacia patellae. The clinical feature is the knee giving way. A tear of a cruciate ligament can cause the knee to give way suddenly without pain and is likely to occur when a runner changes direction suddenly. Instability is classified as straight non-rotatory (which can be anterior, posterior, media or lateral) or rotatory (which can be anteromedial, anterolateral, posterolateral or combined).

See also Pivot shift test

Knee medial ligament strain

Medial ligament strain of the knee can be due, in a contact sport, to a direct valgus force to the outside of the knee or, in skiing, to the foot being stuck on the ski while the leg twists in lateral tibial rotation. It is the most commonly injured of all the knee ligaments. The injury is classified as first degree (mild), second degree (moderate) and third degree (severe).

In *first degree strain* only a few fibres are torn and the ligament does not lose its integrity. Clinical features are pain, tenderness and, sometimes, a small hematoma at the site of the injury. The joint is stable.

In *second degree strain* there is an incomplete tear of the ligament. The pain, tenderness and disability are more severe, but there is no pathological laxity and only slight instability. A blood-stained synovial effusion may be present.

In *third degree strain* there is a complete rupture of the capsular ligament, with the ligament being torn from its upper attachment to the femur. Although the immediate pain and disability are great, the pain eases in time and the patient may be able to walk a little. Synovial fluid may be present, but it can disappear though the tear.

Treatment of a first degree strain involves rest, ice, elevation of the limb and isometric and hip exercises. Treatment of a second degree strain is similar to that for a first degree strain, with the addition of compression to control the swelling. Treatment of a third degree strain is surgical.

Knee meniscal cysts

Meniscal cysts of the knee are far more common in the lateral meniscus than in the medial meniscus. They can follow a blow or a degenerative tear. Synovial fluid can enter the cyst and fill it with a thick gelatinous fluid containing hyaluronic acid. Clinical features are pain, a tender palpable mass and, sometimes, effusion of the joint. The pain is intermittent and made worse by running or climbing stairs. Treatment involves arthroscopy, surgical removal of the cyst and repair of the meniscus.

Knee meniscal injuries

Knee meniscal injuries occur in athletes of all ages, including children. In young athletes a sudden tear of the meniscus can be due to twisting the knee, suddenly changing running direction, squatting forcefully or a contact injury when the knee is struck from the lateral or anterolateral direction. Meniscal tears are often associated with collateral and cruciate ligament injuries. The patient is likely to complain of a tearing or popping sensation in the knee, of the knee locking or giving way and pain in the line of the joint on the side of the torn meniscus; an intra-articular effusion may follow. There can be a reflex inhibition of the quadriceps muscle. In older athletes with degenerated menisci the tear can follow a minor injury or a minor load applied to the knee. In children meniscal tears are rare; they can occur in congenitally abnormal menisci. A tear in the vascular region of the meniscus in a young athlete is likely to heal spontaneously. Other tears are likely to need surgical treatment by partial or complete meniscectomy.

Knee meniscal ossicles

Meniscal ossicles of the knee are small rounded bony structures in the menisci which are either congenital or follow injury to the knee. The symptoms are pain and locking, although they can be asymptomatic. Diagnosis is by X-ray. Treatment is surgical.

L

Laceration

Laceration is a wound of the skin. In athletes it is most likely to occur in the lips, eyebrow region and scalp. Sports in which it is likely to occur are boxing, wrestling, cricket and skiing. Treatment involves compression and, if necessary, irrigation and suturing.

See also facial laceration, scalp laceration

Lachman's test

Lachman's test is a test of the integrity of the anterior cruciate ligament of the knee. It assesses anterior knee laxity and stiffness with the knee in 20° of flexion. An increase in joint laxity and a decrease in end-point stiffness are signs of injury to the ligament.

See also Knee anterior cruciate ligament injury

Laseque's test

Laseque's test determines whether a sciatic nerve root lesion is present by stretching the dura and nerve roots. The patient lies supine with the hip flexed to 90° and the knee is slowly extended until radicular pain is felt. The test is less specific than the straight leg raising test.

Lateral epicondylitis
See Tennis elbow

Lateral hypercompression syndrome
See Patellofemoral pain syndrome

Lateral ligament ankle sprain

Lateral ligament ankle sprain occurs in children and is due to the lateral fibular epiphysis moving out of position and then springing back into position. There is tenderness over the epiphysial line of the fibula. Treatment involves immobilization in plaster.

Latissimus dorsi injury

Latissimus dorsi injury may be a contusion in a contact sport or a sprain in a throwing sport. Clinical features can be tenderness to deep palpation and pain with resistance to adduction of the shoulder. Treatment involves rest from the sport.

Lesser trochanter avulsion

Avulsion of the lesser trochanter can occur due to spasm of the iliopsoas muscle in adolescent players of American football before they have reached full skeletal maturity. Clinical features are pain and spasm of the muscle. Treatment involves rest and positioning to relax iliopsoas until symptom-free; there is a gradual return to full activity. Non-union is a complication which may require surgical excision of the un-united fragment.

Levator scapulae syndrome

Other names Scapulocostal syndrome, scapulothoracic bursitis, superior scapular syndrome

Levator scapulae syndrome is due to tendonitis of the levator scapulae muscle with degeneration of the tendon. It is likely to be produced by repetitive overhead movements of the shoulder. Clinical features are muscular spasm, painful trigger-points and painful palpation. Treatment involves physiotherapy and injection of a local anesthetic.

Little League elbow

Other name Thomas' elbow

Little League elbow occurs in boy baseball pitchers in the Little League; it can also occur in young tennis players. It is an apophysitis of the medial epicondyle. Clinical features are pain and stiffness in the elbow and tenderness over the medial epicondyle.

Treatment involves giving up throwing for up to 8–10 weeks and immobilization of the elbow. Surgery may be necessary if the condition becomes chronic.

Little League shoulder

Little League shoulder is a fatigue fracture or a slip of the epiphyseal plate in the head of the humerus which occurs in boy baseball pitchers playing in Little League. He complains of pain in the shoulder and an inability to pitch. Treatment involves rest either for about 6 weeks, until the symptoms disappear or until healing appears on X-rays.

Low back injuries

Low back injuries can occur in wrestling, usually as sprains and strains. Fracture of the lumbar spine and disc herniation are very uncommon. The wrestler is likely to complain of pain and a feeling of something twisting in his or her back. The pain may disappear within a week or two or persist for months. Treatment involves rest from wrestling, ice, non-steroidal anti-inflammatory drugs, transcutaneous nerve stimulation and flexibility and strengthening exercises.

Lumbar disc degeneration and herniation

Lumbar disc *degeneration* is common in older athletes. Clinical features are low back pain which is aggravated by exercise, muscle spasm which flattens the lumbar contour and tenderness on percussion in the midline. Treatment involves exercises to strengthen the paraspinal and abdominal muscles, moist heat and massage to relieve pain and spasm, and wearing an elastic brace.

Lumbar disc *herniation* can occur while an athlete is engaged in sport or shortly afterwards. He or she may feel a 'pop' or 'snap' in the back, which is followed by pain in the buttocks and legs. This can be associated with either (a) compression of a nerve root causing weakness and numbness in a leg; or (b) compression of the cauda equina producing bilateral leg weakness and numbness, incontinence or retention. Initial treatment involves rest and analgesics. If this does not improve the condition with 7 days, corticosteroid and narcotics can be injected into the epidural space. Surgery may be necessary if the response to other treatment is unsatisfactory.

Lumbar disc herniation
See Lumbar disc degeneration and herniation

Lumbar spine injuries

Lumbar spine injuries can be soft tissue injuries, lumbar spine fracture or fracture/dislocation of the lumbar spine.

Soft tissue injuries can cause musculoligamentous strain with low back pain and muscle spasm, which in the older athlete can be associated with degenerative changes in the vertebrae. Treatment involves cold therapy to reduce edema and inflammation, wearing a lumbosacral corset and rehabilitation exercises.

Lumbar spine fracture is uncommon in athletes. It can be (a) a compression fracture of a vertebral body; or (b) a fracture of a spinous or transverse process. The patient will give a history of trauma and complain of severe pain over the fracture. Compression fracture of a vertebral body can be associated with cauda equina injury, and so the patient should be questioned about any numbness, weakness or pain in the legs. Fracture of a transverse or spinous process can be due to a direct blow from, for example, an American football helmet, and can be associated with renal damage, as can be demonstrated by hematuria. If there is any evidence or threat of neurological damage the patient should be immobilized and moved with a spine scoop and board. Treatment of a compression fracture involves immobilization in a thoracolumbar orthosis for 4–6 weeks for a young athlete and up to 12 weeks for an older adult, followed by rehabilitation exercises; surgery may be necessary for severe compression injury. Treatment of a transverse or spinous process fracture is by cold therapy, analgesics and immobilization in a brace or corset.

Fracture/dislocation of the lumbar spine is a very rare sports injury and can be produced only by very severe force. One vertebra is dislocated over another. The cauda equina is likely to be damaged. Surgical treatment is necessary.

Maisoneuve fracture

Maisoneuve fracture is a fracture of the proximal fibular shaft which may occur in combination with an ankle injury due to pronation/external rotation of the foot.

Mallet finger

Other names Baseball finger, drop finger, hammer finger

Mallet finger is due to the avulsion of an extensor tendon. It is most likely to occur in football, basketball, baseball and cricket players when they catch a ball. It is due to acute flexion of the distal interphalangeal joint. There may be avulsion of a small speck of bone from the dorsum of the distal phalanx. Treatment involves splinting the distal joint without immobilization of the proximal joint for 6–10 weeks. Surgery may be required.

March hemoglobinuria

March hemoglobinuria can follow prolonged walking or marathon running. It is due to intravascular hemolysis. Clinical features are dark or red urine and sometimes nausea and abdominal pain. The condition is self-limited and does not cause permanent damage.

Martial arts injuries

Martial arts injuries occur mainly to the head, neck, and less frequently on the trunk and limbs. They include concussion, loss of consciousness, post-traumatic encephalopathy, lacerations, hematomas, muscle strains, joint strains, fractured ribs, fractured metacarpals and metatarsals, and dislocated and fractured digits. Factors contributing to injury are inadequate training, inadequate safety equipment, head contact and inadequate medical supervision.

McMurray's test

McMurray's test assesses whether the menisci of the knee are torn and displaced. A displaceable fragment of a torn lateral meniscus can produce pain or a palpable click, usually along the posterolateral joint line, if the fully flexed knee is brought into extension by a combination of external rotation and valgus stretch. A displaceable torn tear of the medial meniscus can produce tenderness along the posteromedial joint line if the hyperflexed knee is extended by a combination of internal rotation and varus stretch.

Medial collateral ligament rupture of the elbow

Medial collateral ligament rupture can occur in baseball pitchers and javelin throwers. The rupture can be preceded by several months or years of mild pain and tenderness at the medial side of the elbow. Rupture causes a sudden pain followed by tenderness and bruising. Treatment involves rest, ice, and non-steroidal anti-inflammatory drugs; surgery may be necessary if the condition has not been cured in six months.

Medial epicondylar stress fracture

Stress fracture of the humeral medial epicondyle can occur in children and adolescents who are baseball pitchers and throwers. In a child a large fragment can be displaced and malrotated; in an adolescent the epicondyle is fragmented but the fracture fragment is small. The patient presents with a painful and swollen elbow, bruising, limitation of movement and tenderness in the epicondyle. Surgical treatment may be required.

Medial epicondylitis
See Golfer's elbow, tennis elbow

Medial malleolar stress fracture

Medial malleolar stress fracture can occur in jumpers and runners who then present with pain, tenderness and swelling. Treatment involves a cast or internal fixation.

Medial tibial stress syndrome

Other name Shin splints

Medial tibial stress syndrome is dull ache, soreness or pain, which can be severe, felt over the posteromedial border of the tibia in the middle and distal thirds of the leg. In runners, especially the untrained and inexperienced, it occurs initially towards the end of the exercise and later throughout the whole exercise and in other activities. Changes in running surface and footwear can be contributing factors. Clinical findings are tenderness along the posterior medial border of the middle and lower thirds of the tibia, and sometimes slight swelling. Treatment involves rest, ice, non-steroidal anti-inflammatory drugs, improvement in technique and proper running shoes. If conservative treatment fails, surgery may be required.

Median nerve compression

Median nerve compression at the elbow usually occurs in weight-lifters and tennis players, but can be due to a blow on the proximal arm in any sport. Clinical features may include aching in the forearm, numbness of the hand and fatigue of the forearm. Treatment involves support for the arm, non-steroidal anti-inflammatory drugs and rehabilitation exercises.

Metacarpal fracture

Fracture of a metacarpal can be transverse or comminuted as the result of a direct blow, or spiral or oblique as the result of a twisting injury. Clinical features are pain, swelling and sometimes deformity. Treatment involves closed reduction and external immobilization. An unstable fracture may require closed reduction and percutaneous pin fixation.

Metatarsal stress fracture

Stress fracture of a metatarsal can occur in runners, jumpers and American football players. It presents with pain, tenderness and swelling. Treatment involves rest from sporting activities and supports until there is no pain.

Metatarsophalangeal joint injuries

Metatarsophalangeal joint injuries can occur in football players who play in lightweight flexible shoes. Another risk factor is playing on an artificial surface. The injury can be either a fracture of the head of the first metatarsal, or a dislocation or strain of the metatarsophalangeal joint (turf toe) due to hyperextension. Stress fracture of one or both of the sesamoid bones of flexor hallucis brevis can be an associated condition. Clinical features vary with the extent of the injury, but pain, tenderness, swelling and hemorrhage are common. Treatment also depends on the severity of the lesion and generally involves compression, ice, non-steroidal anti-inflammatory drugs and taping the toe. Reduce a dislocation immediately. A stiff insole should be worn in the shoe on return to football.

Migraine

An attack of migraine can be precipitated by the stress of competitive sport. An attack is most likely in a person who has had a previous attack, but it can occur in an athlete who has never had one. Clinical features are those of a typical migraine, with prodromal symptoms, an aura, a severe and usually unilateral headache, vomiting, and sometimes an episode of confusion and spatial disorientation. An attack may last for several hours or for up to 3 days. The athlete should rest from training and competitions for several weeks after an attack, but further attacks are likely in subsequent competitions.

Miliaria rubra
See Prickly heat

Milligram's test

Milligram's test assesses sciatic nerve tension. The patient lies supine and raises both legs several centimeters above the table and holds the position for 30 seconds. A positive result is one in which radicular leg pain is reproduced.

Miserable malalignment syndrome

Miserable malalignment syndrome is frequently experienced by runners and involves pain and malfunction of the knee due to a malalignment of the femur and patella. It is more common in women than men because women tend to have a wider pelvis and so a larger Q-angle (this is the angle between a line drawn from the tibial tuberosity vertically upwards through the center of the patella and a line drawn from the center of the patella to the anterior superior iliac spine). There may also be an excessive internal rotation of the femur with secondary external tibial torsion and hyperpronation of the feet. It can be associated with patellofemoral pain syndrome.

See also Patellofemoral pain syndrome

Molluscum contagiosum

Molluscum contagiosum is an infection of the skin by a poxvirus. Athletes most likely to be affected are swimmers and cross-country runners; it can also be transmitted in contact sports, especially wrestling. Clinical features are whitish-yellow, flesh-colored or red papules, sometimes with central umbilication. Histological examination shows characteristic viral inclusions. Treatment can involve topical retinoin (Retin-A), freezing and curetting, or electrodesiccation. An infected person should not engage in contact sports until cured.

Monteggia's fracture/dislocation

Monteggia's fracture/dislocation is a fracture of the ulnar shaft with dislocation of the radial head. It can be due to falling on an outstretched hand. Three types have been described and it is associated with injury to the radial nerve and its posterior interosseous branches, to the ulnar nerve and to the anterior interosseous nerve.

Mountaineering disorders
See High altitude disorders

Multidirectional instability of the shoulder joint

Multidirectional instability of the shoulder joint is instability occurring in more than one plane, the most common forms being (a) anterior dislocation with inferior and posterior subluxation; (b) posterior dislocation with anterior and inferior subluxation; and (c) dislocation in all three directions. It is a complication of inferior capsular laxity, which is likely to occur in swimmers, weight-lifters and throwers, and can be a result of multiple injuries to the joint. Treatment can be conservative or surgical.

Multiple neuritis
See Parsonage–Turner syndrome

Muscle cramp

Muscle cramp is pain in a muscle which occurs during, or immediately after, exercise. It is most common in the gastrocnemius and soleus muscles of the calf and can continue for several days. It can also follow excess sweating and diuresis. The cause is uncertain. It can sometimes be stopped by contraction of an antagonist muscle or by forceful stretching of the affected muscle. Preventive measures include taking adequate fluid and sodium before exercise.

Muscle delayed-onset soreness

Muscle delayed-onset soreness is an aching muscular pain which starts developing several hours after exercise and is likely to be at its most intense 1–2 days later. It is particularly noticeable along fascial or tendinous connections in the muscle. The cause is uncertain, but it may be in connective tissue rather than in muscle fibres.

Muscle pull
See Muscle strain

Muscle rupture
See Muscle strain

Muscle strain

Other names Muscle pull, muscle rupture, muscle tear

Muscle strain is a partial or complete tear of a muscle, usually at the musculotendinous junction, and is generally due to a strong muscular contraction during an excessively powerful muscular stretch. Clinical features are bleeding into the muscle and under the skin, pain and point tenderness. In grade I a small number of muscle fibers is torn without the surrounding fascia being torn. In grade II a large number of muscle fibers are torn, the athlete feels a tearing or popping sensation, and a small defect at the musculotendinous junction may be palpable. In grade III there is complete rupture, with severe pain, loss of function and a palpable defect. Treatment involves rest, ice, compression and immobilization for grades I and II, with oral corticosteroids for grade II. Surgery is required for grade III.

Muscle tear
See Muscle strain

Mycobacterium marinum infection

See Swimming pool granuloma

Myositis ossificans

Myositis ossificans is an ossification developing in a hematoma which is located either in a muscle, at a fracture site or in an injured joint. A common site is attached to the femur near the hip joint; a less common site is the humerus. There is thought to be an osteoblastic invasion from periosteum into the hematoma, for which risk factors are massage and excessive muscular activity. Clinical features are the development of a hard painful mass with restricted movement in the affected muscle and muscle atrophy. The bony mass should slowly regress. Treatment involves rest, analgesics, non-steroidal anti-inflammatory drugs, immobilization, active stretching and strengthening exercises. The patient should be able to return to active sport in 3–4 months and should wear protective padding over the affected area. If surgical removal of the ossified area is necessary, it should be postponed for 12 months by which time active ossification will have ceased.

N

Nail injuries

Finger or toenail injuries can be avulsion or subungual hematoma. Treatment of a hematoma involves drainage by perforating holes with a needle or hot paperclip under digital block. In both conditions an appropriate dressing is applied.

Nasal damage

Damage to the nose can be due to a punch in boxing. Such an injury in a young person may interfere with the normal development of the nose and can cause persistent nasal obstruction. The nasal bones can be fractured and the cartilaginous septum broken into several pieces. Damage to the septum can cause scarring which interferes with an operation to restore an adequate airway and may prevent a good airway being produced.

Navicular accessory bone disorder

An accessory navicular bone is found in 2–14% of people and can be unilateral or bilateral. It develops from a secondary ossification center at the tuberosity of the navicular bone and can fuse with it in adolescence. Usually it is asymptomatic, but it can cause a dull midtarsal aching pain with tenderness at the attachment site of the posterior tibial tendon to the navicular. A bursa can develop over it and become inflamed. The diagnosis is confirmed by X-ray. Treatment involves rest, immobilization in a short leg cast and non-steroidal anti-inflammatory drugs. Surgical excision may be required if conservative treatment has not produced recovery in 6 months.

Navicular stress fracture

Stress fracture of the navicular bone can occur in sprinters, runners, jumpers and American football players. The fracture can be partial or complete and presents with a dull ache, tenderness and swelling in the medial arch area. X-ray may not be diagnostic at first, but a technetium bone scan can be more helpful. Treatment involves plaster immobilization for 6–8 weeks; if the fracture is displaced or non-union occurs surgery is required.

Neuralgic amyotrophy
See Parsonage–Turner syndrome

Non-cardiac syncope

Non-cardiac syncope is a condition most likely to occur in adolescent athletes when they have failed in a competitive event. They collapse, complain of weakness and may appear to be disorientated. The heart is normal. Psychological factors are the causes.

O

Ober's test

Ober's test is a test of iliotibial band tightness. The patient lies on his or her side with the leg to be examined uppermost. The unaffected knee and hip are flexed. The affected knee is then flexed to 90° and the hip is abducted and hyperextended. A tight tibial band prevents the limb from dropping below the horizontal.

Olecranon bursitis

Olecranon bursitis is a common condition in athletes, especially in footballers and hockey players. It can present as an acute condition after a blow on the elbow, becoming swollen and tender, but it can also present as a chronic condition with swelling and indurated walls. Surgery may be necessary. A complication is the development of sepsis in the bursa, which can present with local inflammation, pain and tenderness; the inflammation can spread to the forearm or cause a systemic infection. The diagnosis is confirmed by examination of fluid obtained from the bursa by aspiration. Treatment involves oral antibiotics and the injection of an appropriate antibiotic into the bursa.

Olecranon epiphysial stress fracture

Stress fracture of the olecranon epiphysis can occur in young athletes, who present with pain in the elbow. X-ray may show widening of the epiphysial line. Fusion can occur late or incompletely. Treatment involves immobilization, but if this fails surgery is required to obtain union.

Olecranon osteochondrosis

Osteochondrosis of the olecranon apophysis can present in child athletes with pain, swelling and tenderness of the olecranon. Treatment involves rest and temporary immobilization.

One-ball-left syndrome
See Testicular trauma

Osgood–Schlatter disease

Osgood–Schlatter disease occurs in adolescence as a result of repetitive stress on the patellar tendon at its insertion into the tibial tubercle before the apophysis has united. It is most common in boys aged 10–14 years who engage in running and jumping. The boy complains of a gradual pain localized to the insertion of the infrapatellar tendon into the tibia. Clinical features are a tender swelling over the tibial tubercle, soft tissue swelling in the area, erythema and increased tenderness. With a rest from sporting activities the condition improves slowly, recovery occurring at about 14 years of age when the tibial tubercle apophysis closes. Treatment involves isometric exercises, stretching and passive movements to strengthen the hamstring muscles, and strengthening of the quadriceps muscle. An infrapatellar strap may be worn. Crutches may be necessary for severe and prolonged disability.

Osteitis pubis

Osteitis pubis is a pathological condition of the pubis characterized by bone resorption at the medial ends of the pubis, rarefaction or sclerosis of the rami, and widening of the pubic symphysis. It can occur in athletes. Its cause is unknown. Clinical features are pain in the pubic region radiating into the thigh or abdominal wall, spasm in the adductor or abdominal muscles and, in severe cases, a waddling gait. The condition may be self-limited, but may persist for several months. Treatment involves rest and non-steroidal anti-inflammatory drugs. Surgery can include local debridement or arthrodesis of the pubic symphysis for chronic osteitis pubis which has not responded to a more conservative approach.

Osteoarthritis of the knee

Osteoarthritis of the knee is a common late complication of any knee injury in sports people. Clinical features are slowly developing discomfort, stiffness and limitation of movement. Treatment involves rest, reduction of weight, non-steroidal anti-inflammatory drugs, knee support, strengthening exercises for the quadriceps muscle and passive mobilization.

Osteochondritis dissecans

Osteochondritis is a condition which affects either the knee or the talus and involves separation (partial or complete) of hyaline cartilage from its supporting bone. Although it is most likely to present in the twenties, it can occur in childhood.

Osteochondritis of the knee is thought to be due to trauma, but it can occur after twisting injuries and it has also been attributed to ischemia and anomalies of ossification. It is characterized by degeneration or aseptic necrosis and recalcification. If the hyaline cartilage remains partly attached, clinical features are a swollen knee and dull pain which is present both day and night and made worse by exercise. If the cartilage is completely detached, locking, catching or giving way of the knee can occur. The quadriceps muscle is likely to be weakened or atrophic. Treatment involves rest and avoidance of weight-bearing. If a loose body is present, surgical removal is necessary.

Osteochondritis of the talus is pathologically similar to osteochondritis of the knee and can be lateral or medial. The patient is likely to complain of a sprained ankle. There may be locking or giving way of the joint. Treatment is conservative at first, with surgery being necessary to remove a loose body.

Osteoporosis

Osteoporosis is a loss of mineral density in bone. The mineral density of bone is controlled by several factors which include genetics, diet (especially calcium intake), estrogen, menstrual status and physical activity. Exercise increases the density, with the effect tending to be localized to the part of the body under the greatest stress. Gravity is a stress stimulus and weight-bearing sports have a greater effect than non-weight-bearing sports such as swimming. Intensive aerobic training can have an adverse effect on bone density by suppressing ovarian function, which leads to a reduction in estrogen levels, one result of which is amenorrhea. Psychological stress may play a part in the process.

Women with low levels of estrogen show a reduction in bone density level. In menstruating women bone density level tends to increase up to about 35 years of age, and then declines slowly until the time of the menopause, after which there is a rapid loss for 5–10 years. Most women cross the 'fracture level' (the degree of bone density below which fractures can be due to minor trauma) at about 65 years. An athlete who has been amenorrheal in her twenties and thirties may not achieve normal bone density; she is also likely to start losing bone density at 35 years and to cross the 'fracture threshold' at a much earlier age than a woman who menstruated normally. The more intensely a girl or young women trains the more likely she is to develop amenorrhea and osteoporosis with its risk of fractures.

Overtraining syndrome
See Burnout

Overuse injuries

Overuse injuries are endemic in sport due to the pressure to succeed; the desire of amateurs to achieve professional standards, overtraining, stress, and parents pressurizing their children. They are particularly liable to occur in adolescents who are devoted to a single sport, have a high level of commitment, boast about their toughness, are always trying too hard and are repeatedly asking for their coach's approval. Contributing factors are too great a training and exercise load, poor technique, faulty posture and limb alignment, and faulty equipment. Tissues likely to develop overuse injuries are joints (leading to pain, tenderness, effusion and restriction of movement), bone (leading to stress fractures, shin soreness and metabolic overactivity revealed by technetium scanning) and ligaments (leading to overstrain). Preventive measures include advice from a coach and parents, identifying possible causes, taking time off and relaxing, correcting poor technique, training to acceptable levels, replacement of bad equipment with good, stretching and warm up before engaging in a sport, and, in children, adequate supervision and reduction of pressure. Treatment involves rest, either general or sport-specific, ice on the affected parts, non-steroidal anti-inflammatory drugs and a gradual progression from low-level training to full training.

See also Burnout

P

Paget–von Schrötter syndrome
See Effort thrombosis

Painful subacromial arc syndrome

Painful subacromial arc syndrome is characterized by severe pain during only a part of active excursion of the shoulder, with full painless passive movement. The pain is felt in the deltoid muscle, is sometimes felt in the shoulder region, can radiate down the arm and is severe at night. Radiography may show a normal shoulder or degeneration in the acromioclavicular joint and the greater tuberosity of the humerus. In some patients the .pain abates spontaneously after a few weeks; in others it becomes chronic.

Pain measurement

Pain is a common symptom of injury and objective methods of measuring it have been devised in order to assess the progress and the effectiveness of treatments. It can be measured by rating scales, questionnaires and indirect methods.

Rating scales are simple and easy to administer. The ones usually used are binary scales, categorical verbal rating scales, visual analog scales and verbal scales. Binary scales are designed to produce a yes or no answer to a question. In a categorical verbal rating scale (or categorical scale) the patient is shown a list of descriptions and is asked to choose the one which most appropriately describes what he or she is feeling. With a visual analog scale the patient is shown a series of 10 cm lines whose ends are labelled with extreme descriptions (such as 'No relief of pain' at one end and 'Complete relief of pain' at the other) and asked to mark where along the line he or she feels his or her condition lies. With a verbal numerical scale the patient provides his or her assessment as a number on a 11-point scale.

The usual *questionnaires* used are the Wisconsin Brief Pain Questionnaire and the McGill Pain Questionnaire. They take longer to administer than scales, but they have the advantage of being a multidimensional measure of pain, covering such aspects as the effects on activities, sleep and mood.

Indirect measurements of pain are by pulse, blood pressure, respiratory rate, skin temperature, electroencephalogram (EEG) and evoked potentials, but none of these are very reliable. Another indirect method is by the number of doses of analgesic requested by the patient.

Palpitations

In athletes palpitations may occur during exercise and not at other times. An electrocardiogram (ECG) may show arrhythmias which may be caused by supraventricular tachycardia.

Pancreatitis

Pancreatitis can be due to an upper abdominal blow which can occur in American football, karate, football and skiing. Clinical features are severe upper abdominal pain and tenderness. Serum amylase is raised. Complications are hemorrhage, a pseudocyst, an abscess of the pancreas, and hematoma and rupture of the duodenum.

Paroxysmal nocturnal hemoglobinuria

Paroxysmal nocturnal hemoglobinuria is an acquired hemolytic disorder associated with increased susceptibility of a red cell subpopulation to mediated damage. It usually occurs during sleep, but it can follow severe exercise. Clinical features are dark urine (containing hemoglobin), back pain, iron deficiency and a liability to develop venous thromboses.

Par-Q test

Other name Physical activity readiness questionnaire

The Par-Q test is designed to detect those athletes in whom physical activity is likely to induce heart diseases. The modified version is shown in Table 7.

Table 7 A modified version of the PAR-Q test which is designed to detect athletes in whom physical exercise is likely to induce heart disease

1. Are you over 60 years of age?	Yes/No
2. Do you suffer from chest pains?	Yes/No
3. Do you suffer from breathlessness or dizziness?	Yes/No
4. Are you a diabetic?	Yes/No
5. Do you have a heart condition or heart murmur or have you had cardiac surgery?	Yes/No
6. Have you been told you have a high blood pressure?	Yes/No
7. Do you smoke?	Yes/No
8. Have you suffered from blackouts?	Yes/No

Parsonage–Turner syndrome

Other names Acute brachial neuropathy, brachial plexus neuropathy, multiple neuritis, neuralgic amyotrophy

Parsonage–Turner syndrome can occur in athletes and non-athletes. Its cause is unknown, but it has been attributed to viral infections and allergies. Clinical features include an acute burning pain in the dominant arm which begins in the shoulder girdle and spreads down the arm. The pain resolves in about 2 weeks and is followed by neuritis of the long thoracic, axillary, anterior interosseous, suprascapular and musculocutaneous nerves, as well as atrophy of the deltoid, supraspinatus, infraspinatus and serratus anterior muscles. Paralysis of the serratus anterior causes winging of the scapula. Sensation is not usually markedly affected. Treatment involves analgesics, a sling and rehabilitation of affected muscles when the pain has subsided. Functional recovery can take up to 3 years, although some permanent weakness often persists.

Passive patellar tilt test

Passive patellar tilt test assesses the relationship of the patella to the femur. The patient lies prone with the knee in full extension and the quadriceps relaxed. The examiner stands at the foot of the table and presses posteriorly on the medial edge of the patella to elevate its lateral edge from the lateral femoral condyle with the patella remaining in the trochlea and not being allowed to subluxate. If an excessively tight lateral restraint is present it will not allow the patella to reach the neutral or horizontal position.

Patellar dislocation

Dislocation of the patella can be due to a twisting injury with strong contraction of the quadriceps muscle. It hardly ever occurs in a normal knee, but it is likely to occur when the extensor mechanism is malaligned, the patella misplaced, there is vastus lateralis imbalance or an abnormal Q angle (for a definition of Q angle see page 86). The athlete feels the dislocation and collapse of the knee and is likely to fall to the ground. When it occurs the knee is locked in flexion, the patella can be felt lying laterally, the medial retinaculum is swollen and tender, and there may be a hemarthrosis. An osteochondral fracture can be a complication. Treatment involves reduction, elevation, ice and immobilization; a large hemarthrosis needs to be aspirated. Athroscopic surgery may be required to remove an osteochondrial fragment.

Patellar fracture

Patellar fracture can be due to falling on a hard surface or some other direct blow to the front of the knee; rarely it is due to a violent contracture of the quadriceps muscle. Clinical features of an undisplaced fracture are tenderness, painful movement of the knee and swelling due to an effusion. With a displaced fracture there is disruption of the patella and retinaculum. Treatment of an undisplaced fracture involves immobilization with an early return to mobility. A displaced fracture requires surgery.

Patellar mobility tests

Patellar mobility tests are the Carson test, the Kolwich test, the apprehension test and the tilt test.

Carson test: the patella should displace medially or laterally no more than half the width of the patella. Further displacement suggests that there is excessive retinacular laxity.

Kolwich test: the patella is divided into four longitudinal quadrants and is held between thumb and index finger. Medial displacement of one quadrant suggests a tight retinaculum. Medial displacement of three to four quadrants suggests a hypermobile patella without tightness of lateral restraints. Lateral displacement of three quadrants suggests an incompetent medial restraint. Lateral displacement of four quadrants indicates a dislocatable patella.

Apprehension test: if the patient has had a recent acute subluxation or dislocation of the patella or has chronic hypermobility of the patella, with displacement of the patella laterally, he or she experiences acute discomfort and apprehension.

Tilt test: this evaluates the position of the inferior pole of the patella relative to the superior pole. On contraction of quadriceps muscle, if the inferior pole tilts posteriorly compared to the superior pole, a sharp pain can be felt medial to the patellar tendon as it digs into the infrapatellar fatty pad.

Patellar osteochondritis dissecans
See Sindig–Larsen–Johannson syndrome

Patellar subluxation

Subluxation (an incomplete or partial dislocation) of the patella can occur in sport, with the athlete reporting that the kneecap slipped when he pivoted, cut or twisted. Risk factors are an extensor mechanism malalignment and a previous dislocation. Clinical features are tenderness in the anterior aspect of the knee, swelling due to an effusion and hypermobility of the patella. Treatment can be conservative with muscle-strengthening exercises, muscle re-education, non-steroidal anti-inflammatory drugs and patellofemoral bracing. Surgery may be necessary if these fail.

Patellar tendonitis

Patellar tendonitis can develop in runners, footballers and athletes who engage in lower extremity weight-lifting. Risk factors are running up a steep hill, isotonic knee extension exercises with weights and repetitions of deep knee bends. The clinical feature is pain on going up and down stairs, on rising from the sitting position and on squatting. Treatment involves rest, ice, non-steroidal anti-inflammatory drugs and wearing a knee brace with a patellar insert to prevent lateral patellar tracking.

See also Jumper's knee

Patellar tendon rupture

Rupture of the patellar tendon can occur in weight-lifting and other sports in which great strain is placed on the tendon. Risk factors are jumper's knee, patellar tendonitis, previous steroid injection into the tendon and autoimmune disease. The athlete feels a sudden 'pop' and cannot support any weight on the leg.

Clinical features are a swollen knee, tenderness at the upper or lower pole of the patella and proximal or distal displacement of the patella. Flexing the knee causes patella baja (the patella being lower than in its normal position). Treatment is surgical.

Patellofemoral malalignment syndrome

Patellofemoral malalignment syndrome usually occurs in adolescents and competitive female runners, and less frequently in basketball players, jumpers and cyclists. A wide pelvis increases the lateral pull on the patella during leg extension. Clinical features are discomfort or pain during exercise and on climbing stairs, subluxation of the patella when jumping or climbing, tenderness at the superolateral or inferomedial poles and in the infrapatellar tendon, and sometimes crepitus. Treatment involves wearing appropriate supporting shoes.

Patellofemoral pain syndrome

Other names Chondromalacia patellae, excessive lateral hypercompression syndrome, lateral hypercompression syndrome

Patellofemoral pain syndrome is pain around the extensor mechanism of the knee without evidence of patellofemoral instability. The causes are uncertain, but it has been attributed to chondromalacia patellae (a degeneration of the patellar cartilage), excessive pressure on the lateral part of the patellofemoral joint, stretched ligaments, stretched medial retinaculum, traumatic synovitis and abnormal timing in firing of the components which make the quadriceps muscle. The patient complains of pain in the anterior aspect of one or both knees. The pain may follow a blow to the part or arise spontaneously; it is made worse by exercise and relieved by rest. There may be contracture of the quadriceps muscle, the hamstrings, gastrocnemius, soleus and the iliotibial band. Extensor mechanism malalignment is present. Treatment varies according to what is believed to be the cause of the condition. Recommended are muscle-strengthening exercises, muscle re-education, techniques using electromyographic (EMG) biofeedback, flexibility exercises, patellofemoral bracing and non-steroidal anti-inflammatory drugs. If these fail, an arthroscopic examination of the knee can be performed to identify a possible cause.

Pectoralis major rupture

Pectoralis major rupture is a rare injury which can ocur in male athletes engaged in weight-lifting, rugby, wrestling and strength-training exercises. The rupture can be partial or complete; avulsion of the tendon can occur. Clinical features are severe pain, a tearing sensation, loss of power, bruising and swelling. Partial ruptures are treated with immobilization in a sling and ice, followed by strengthening exercises. Complete tears, although they may be treated conservatively, tend to require surgery; this is also the case for avulsion of the tendon.

Pellegrini–Stieda disease

Pellegrini–Stieda disease is characterized by pain in the medial side of the knee, knee stiffness and a tender lump on the medial condyle of the femur. It can follow a sprain or a direct blow and is most likely to occur in body-contact sports. A hematoma forms in the upper attachment of the medial collateral ligament and can procede to ossification. Treatment involves injection of a corticosteroid and a local anesthetic (which can be repeated at monthly intervals), and by ultrasound, isometric exercises, and later by mobilizing exercises.

Pelvic bone fractures

Fractures of the pelvic bone are severe injuries which can involve the intestines, the genitourinary system and serious blood loss. It can be an avulsion fracture, a pelvic ring fracture and stress fracture of the pubic ramus. Destot's sign, Roux's sign and Earle's sign may be positive.

Avulsion of the lesser trochanter usually occurs in athletes under 20 years of age, is likely to happen while running and is due to an acute sudden contraction of the iliopsoas muscle. The patient complains of a severe anteromedial pain in the hip. The diagnosis is confirmed by X-ray. Treatment involves bed rest followed by rehabilitation exercises. The patient can usually return to full activity in 6–8 weeks.

Fracture of the pelvic rim has occurred in football, hockey, hang-gliding, cycling and horseback riding. Considerable force is required to produce this fracture, and the patient is liable to have severe blood loss, intestinal or vesical damage and soft tissue injuries. Such a fracture usually requires surgical treatment by open reduction, external fixation or internal fixation.

Stress fracture of the pubic ramus can occur in joggers, distance runners and other athletes. The patient complains of pain and is unable to stand unsupported on the affected leg. Treatment involves rest and not running. He or she should be able to return to full activity in 3–5 months.

Pelvic soft tissue contusion

Soft tissue contusion around the pelvis is usually due to a direct blow, such as collision with the playing surface, collision with another player or collision with an American football helmet. The patient complains of pain in the injured area. Most lesions are mild and heal quickly, but slow bleeding can occur in the area leading to subperiosteal hematomas. Treatment is directed at controlling the bleeding by rest, pressure and ice. Myositis ossificans can be a complication of a large intramuscular hematoma.

Peritalar dislocation

Other names Subastragalar dislocation, subtalar dislocation

Peritalar dislocation is dislocation of the talocalcaneal and talonavicular joints due to severe trauma to the ankle. It is usually a medial dislocation; lateral, anterior and posterior dislocations are uncommon. Clinical features are pain, swelling and limitation of movement. Treatment involves immediate reduction (closed or open) followed by a period of immobilization.

Peroneal tendon dislocation

Peroneal tendon dislocation can occur in skiers in a forward fall, when forced dorsiflexion of the ankle causes lengthening of the tendons in the groove posterior to the fibula. The tendons become dislocated from the groove as the peroneal retinaculum and the periosteum on the lateral aspect of the fibular are torn off the lateral malleolus.

Peroneal tendonitis

Peroneal tendonitis can occur in runners and presents as chronic or recurrent pain, swelling and tenderness in the peroneal tendon sheath between the inferior tip of the lateral malleolus and the insertion of peroneus brevis into the base of the fifth metatarsal. Treatment involves rest from running, placing a 1-cm heel lift in the shoe and non-steroidal anti-inflammatory drugs.

Peroneal tendon subluxation

Subluxation of the peroneal tendons generally occurs in skiing, ice-skating, American football, soccer, basketball, but can happen in other sports. The athlete feels a snapping sensation or 'pop' at the ankle posterolaterally and an intense pain which in time subsides to become mild. Clinical examination may reveal swelling over and posterior to the lateral malleolus and the displacement of the tendons may be seen or felt. Acute symptoms may subside quickly and the patient may not seek advice until the condition has become chronic. Acute injuries can be treated conservatively by immobilization in the first instance, but if this fails, and for chronic and repeated subluxation, surgery is necessary.

Pes anserinus bursitis

Pes anserinus bursitus can be due to a direct blow or repeated friction of the pes anserinus bursa, which is situated between the medial collateral ligament of the knee and the pes anserinus (this is the tendinous insertion of the sartorius, gracilis and semi-tendinosus muscles). Clinical features are localized pain, swelling and crepitus. The condition can become chronic if there is a premature return to sporting activities. Treatment involves rest, anti-inflammatory drugs, corticosteroid injection and isometric and resistance exercises.

Phalangeal fracture

Fracture of a phalanx can be transverse or comminuted as the result of a direct blow, or spiral or oblique as the result of a twisting injury. Clinical features are pain, swelling and sometimes deformity. Treatment involves closed reduction and external immobilization. An unstable fracture may require closed reduction and percutaneous pin fixation.

Phalen's test

Phalen's test is a maneuver which assesses whether carpal tunnel syndrome is present. The patient's wrist is placed in unforced complete flexion for 60 seconds. A patient with carpal tunnel syndrome complains of hypoesthesia (decreased sensitivity to stimuli) or paresthesia in the cutaneous distribution of the median nerve in the hand.

Physical activity readiness questionnaire
See PAR-Q test

Piezogenic papules

Piezogenic papules are soft, flesh-colored, uncomfortable papules which are herniations of fat through the connective tissues of the skin of the foot. The papules tend to disappear when the foot is not weight-bearing. Obesity is a contributing factor. Women are more commonly affected than men. Sports which involve jumping should be avoided and support stockings worn.

Ping-pong player purpura

Ping-pong player purpura is the presence of annular purpuric spots on the arms and abdominal wall of a ping-pong player hit by balls travelling at high speed.

Pisiform fracture

Pisiform fracture is due to a direct blow to the palm. Clinical features are pain and tenderness over the base of the hypothenar eminence. Treatment involves immobilization for 3–6 weeks.

Pitted keratolysis

Pitted keratolysis is a bacterial infection of the skin which presents with dents or pits in the stratum corneum, usually in the skin of the soles in athletes. Infecting organisms are likely to be *Streptomyces* sp., *Corynebacterium minutissimum* and *Dermatophilus congolensis*. Excessive sweating is an important factor. Treatment involves the use of drying agents.

Pivot shift test

Pivot shift test is a maneuver which assesses the stability of the knee. The patient lies supine with the hip flexed to 45° and the knee flexed to 90°. The foot is held and rotated medially to its full extent. Valgus stress is applied to the proximal end of the tibia and the knee is gradually extended. If instability of the knee is present, at about 30° of flexion the lateral tibiofemoral compartment will be felt to sublux forwards. With further extension of the knee the tibia will return to its previous position.

Plantar fasciitis
See Heel-spur syndrome

Plica syndrome

Plica syndrome is peripatellar discomfort or pain, clicking or snapping occurring after trauma and due to inflammation or fibrosis of the plica (a congenital synovial septum of the knee) which may be medial, lateral, suprapatellar or infrapatellar. Treatment involves rest, ice, non-steroidal anti-inflammatory drugs and muscle strengthening exercises. Arthroscopic resection of the plica may be necessary.

Popliteal artery entrapment

Popliteal artery entrapment can occur in an athlete who has a congenital anatomic variation of the artery's relationship to gastrocnemius muscle. There are several of these variations, which can be bilateral. The entrapment can cause thrombosis in the artery. Clinical features are paresthesiase, coolness, intermittent claudication, an absent pulse and mild calf tenderness on examination. Arteriography provides a definite diagnosis. Treatment is surgical.

Popliteal tendonitis

Popliteal tendonitis can occur in distance runners and walkers. The onset is usually gradual. The athlete is likely to complain of pain which begins after he or she has run a few miles. The pain is localized over the insertion of the tendon of popliteus into the lateral femoral condyle. The tendon may slip out of and into its groove with a painful click. Clinical features are tenderness at the insertion of the tendon or anterior to the lateral collateral ligament and pain reproduced by contraction of popliteus. Treatment involves rest, non-steroidal anti-inflammatory drugs and modification of running and walking techniques. Local steroid injection may be necessary if the condition does not respond to these measures.

Postconcussive syndrome

Postconcussive syndrome is a complication of concussion and is characterized by persistent headache, irritability, inability to concentrate, fatigue, dizziness, double vision and behavioral disorder which can last for weeks or months after concussion. An athlete should not engage in sport while he or she has any of these features or they are likely to return in full. No treatment is known to speed recovery.

107

Posterior cruciate ligament of the knee tear

Tear of the posterior cruciate ligament of the knee, which is much less common than tear of the anterior cruciate ligament, occurs most frequently in runners and American football players. It is usually associated with other injuries to the knee and can be due to either a twisting strain from a valgus or varus force, falling on the knee with it flexed, or to be hyperflexion without a posteriorly directed force from the ground. Clinical features are retropatellar pain, knee instability, a positive sag sign of Godfrey (the tibia visibly sags backwards on the femur), a positive quadriceps active drawer test and, sometimes, a positive posterior drawer test. Treatment is usually surgical, but can at first be conservative with immobilization and rehabilitation exercises.

Posterior drawer test of the knee

Posterior drawer test is a maneuver which assesses whether there is a tear in the posterior cruciate ligament of the knee. With the patient lying supine, the knee is flexed to 70–90° and the tibia is passively subluxated on the femur. Excessive movement is a positive test. However, as it is not always positive when a tear is present, the quadriceps active drawer test is preferred.

See also Anterior drawer test of the knee, quadriceps active drawer test

Posterior interosseous syndrome

Posterior interosseous syndrome can occur in some athletes, noticeably weight-lifters and bowlers. It is characterized by soreness and aching in the proximal part of the extensor muscle group distal to the lateral epicondyle and is due to the radial nerve being compressed under a fibrous arch at the proximal end of the supinator muscle. There may also be weakness or paralysis of the extensor carpi ulnaris, the thumb adductor and the thumb and finger extensors.

See also Distal posterior interosseous syndrome

Posterior tibialis tendon anterior dislocation

Dislocation of the tendon of the tibialis posterior muscle has occurred in runners. Clinical features were locking of the joint, pain at the medial malleolus and painful eversion and inversion. Treatment is surgical.

Posterior tibial tendonitis

Posterior tibial tendonitis occurs in runners and players of basketball and volleyball, tends to occur in older athletes and is precipitated by a powerful push-off. Clinical features are pain and tenderness behind the medial malleolus, radiating into the calf and distally to the navicular bone, sometimes a palpable swelling of the tendon, and an inability to run properly. Treatment involves rest, non-steroidal anti-inflammatory drugs and raising the medial heel with an arch support. Surgical treatment may be necessary if conservative treatment is ineffective.

Post-traumatic amnesia

Post-traumatic amnesia is the time taken for continuous memory to return after a period of unconsciousness due to brain injury. It is usually three times longer than the length of unconsciousness, but does become longer with age. A period of less than 1 hour indicates a mild head injury; 1–24 hours indicates a moderate injury.

Prepatellar bursitis

Prepatellar bursitis is most likely to occur in footballers, wrestlers and gymnasts. An acute prepatellar bursitis can follow a single blow; clinical features are swelling of the bursa, discomfort or pain, erythema, warmth and crepitation. Chronic or recurrent prepatellar bursitis is due to repeated blows; clinical features are a large painful bursa with thickening of its wall and loculation. Treatment involves immobolization, compression, non-steroidal anti-inflammatory drugs, isometric exercises of quadriceps to prevent atrophy of the muscle, and protective padding when engaged in sport. Surgical removal of a chronic or recurrent bursitis may be necessary.

Prickly heat

Other name Heat rash, miliaria rubra

Prickly heat is characterized by small red prickly papules and vesicles which develop in the skin due to obstruction of sweat glands. It can occur in athletes training or competing in hot humid conditions. The condition is usually self-limiting.

Profundus tendon avulsion
See Jersey finger

Pronator teres syndrome

Pronator teres syndrome is an entrapment of the median nerve at the elbow where it passes between the two heads of pronator teres. It can be due to weight-lifting or underarm, fast ball pitching. Clinical features are likely to be a vague pain in the front of the forearm, pain made worse by athletic exercise, weakness in the palmar flexors of the hand and reduced sensitivity in the radial three and a half digits of the hand. Conservative treatment involves rest, heat and immobilization, but surgery is necessary if these measures fail.

Proximal humeral epiphysiolysis

Proximal humeral epiphysiolysis is a traction injury of the proximal humeral epiphysis which occurs in adolescent baseball pitchers and is characterized by a severe throbbing pain in the shoulder. X-ray shows a widened epiphysial plate. Treatment involves rest from pitching and other exercises causing the pain.

Proximal interphalangeal joint subluxation and dislocation

Proximal interphalangeal joint subluxation and dislocation may be dorsal, volar or rotatory.

Dorsal dislocation can be associated with detachment of a chip of bone from the volar base of the middle phalanx, leading to a painful and swollen finger. The player or coach may reduce the dislocation on the spot, but further treatment will be needed and this involves immobilization for 3–6 weeks. Scar tissue developing at the site can cause a flexion contracture (pseudoboutonnière deformity).

Volar dislocation is very rare and should be treated by reduction and splinting for 3–4 weeks. Surgery may be necessary.

Rotatory dislocation is also rare. It is the result of twisting the finger violently and may require reduction under digital block anesthesia followed by taping.

Pubic bone stress fracture

Stress fracture of the pubic bone can occur in joggers and long distance runners. As with other stress fractures there is a higher incidence in women than in men. Clinical features are pain, tenderness and a positive standing sign (pain or an inability to stand on the affected leg). Treatment involves ceasing to participate in sporting activities until fully recovered.

Punch-drunk syndrome

Other name Dementia pugilistica

Punch-drunk syndrome is likely to occur in professional boxers after about 20 fights and is due to blows to the head or to falls onto the canvas. It is also seen in jockeys who fall frequently. Clinical features are those of a progressive dementia, with impaired intellectual function, memory impairment, morbid jealousy, rage reactions, dysarthria, fits and signs of extrapyramidal and cerebellar degeneration. Pneumoencephalography is likely to show cerebral atrophy and an enlarged cavity of the septum pellucidum.

Q

Quadriceps active drawer test

Quadriceps active drawer test is a maneuver to assess whether there is a tear in the posterior cruciate ligament of the knee. With the patient lying supine, the leg is relaxed and supported by one hand of the examiner with the knee flexed to 90°. The examiner's other hand stabilizes the foot on the couch. The patient is then asked to slide the foot gently down the table. A visible displacement of the tibia anteriorly due to the contraction of the quadriceps muscle is a positive test indicating that the ligament is torn.

Quadriceps muscle contusion

Other name Charley horse

Quadriceps muscle contusion is usually due to a direct injury in a contact sport, often by another player's knee. Muscle fibers are damaged and an intramuscular hematoma is likely to form. The patient complains of pain, tenderness and difficulty in walking. Treatment can involve rest, ice and an early return to gentle movement. Early immobilization in 120° of knee flexion for 24 hours after the injury is said to have better results. Exercise in a swimming pool or whirlpool is helpful. Oral non-steroidal anti-inflammatory drugs and analgesics can be given for severe pain. A possible complication is myositis ossificans.

Quadriceps strain

Quadriceps strain is due to a strong contraction or forceful stretching of the muscle and can occur anywhere along its musculotendinous unit. It is most likely to occur in football and basketball players and in field and track athletes. The person will complain of a severe localized pain in the muscle that is made worse by contraction. Clinical findings can include a localized swelling and loss of flexion at the knee. Treatment involves rest, ice, compression, elevation and non-steroidal anti-inflammatory drugs, followed by exercises and a gradual return to training.

Quadriceps tendonitis

Quadriceps tendonitis is due to excessive strain on the quadriceps tendon. The athlete complains of an aching pain at the insertion of the tendon into the patella that begins insidiously during training. Clinical features are tenderness at the site, tightness of the hamstring muscles and pain on resisted extension of the knee. Treatment involves rest, non-steroidal anti-inflammatory drugs and rehabilitative exercises.

Quadriceps tendon rupture

Quadriceps tendon rupture can be partial or complete. Risk factors are autoimmune disease, jumper's knee and increasing age. It is said that a healthy tendon never ruptures. The athlete may have the sensation of a 'pop'. With a complete rupture there is immediate disability and an inability to stand on the leg; a gap in the tendon may be palpable. A partial tear is treated conservatively by rest, ice and immobilization. A complete tear requires surgery.

Quadrilateral space syndrome

The quadrilateral space is bounded above by teres minor, below by teres major, laterally by the shaft of the humerus and medially by the long head of biceps. The axillary nerve and the posterior humeral circumflex artery pierce the fascial lane between teres major and teres minor and supply teres minor and deltoid. The syndrome occurs in adults aged 20–25 years, and in athletes in the dominant arm. Clinical features are slow intermittent pain and paresthesiae in the upper arm, a painful spot at about the insertion of teres minor and weak extension of the arm. The pain is made worse by throwing movements and can be severe at night. It can be produced by abduction and external rotation of the arm for 1 minute. Arteriogram of the subclavian artery can show that the posterior circumflex artery is patent with the arm at the side and occluded when it is abducted. Treatment involves strengthening the shoulder muscles and avoiding abduction and external rotation of the arm as much as possible. Surgical decompression of the quadrilateral space may be necessary.

R

Reflex sympathetic dystrophy of the knee

Reflex sympathetic dystrophy of the knee is a response of the knee out of proportion to the severity of the injury causing it. Clinical features are pain in various positions about the knee and at night, diffuse swelling, loss of full mobility, muscle wasting, cyanosis of the skin and decreased temperature of the affected leg.

Retrocalcaneal bursitis

Other name Haglund's syndrome

Retrocalcaneal bursitis is an inflammation of the retrocalcaneal bursa, an adventitious bursa situated between the Achilles tendon and the superior tuberosity of the calcaneous. Risk factors are long-distance running, Achilles tendonitis or calcification, ill-fitting or inappropriate shoes, and running on hard surfaces. The patient complains of a dull aching pain, which may have been precipitated by trauma to the tendon or heel. Clinical findings are a swelling between tendon and bone; fluid can occasionally be felt in the bursa. Treatment is conservative, involving a rest from running, wearing well-fitting shoes, running on a soft surface and the injection of corticosteroid into the bursa. If these measures fail, surgery is required.

Retropatellar dysfunction
See Retropatellar pain syndrome

Retropatellar pain syndrome

Other name Retropatellar dysfunction

Retropatellar pain syndrome is pain in the patellar region and tightness of the iliotibial band, the hamstrings, the gastrocnemius muscle and the lateral retinaculum due to an interference with normal patellofemoral movements. It is caused by a mal-alignment of the patella with the intercondylar surface of the femur. There is an altered Q angle (for definition of Q angle see page 86). There may be prolonged or excessive pronation of the subtalar joint which can result in an increase in the Q angle. It can occur in any type of athlete as most sporting activities require a full range of normal patellofemoral movements, and is not a result of a single incidence but due to overuse. Clinical features are likely to be pain and tightening of the iliotibial band, the hamstring muscles, gastrocnemius muscle and the lateral retinaculum. Treatment should be conservative at first, involving rest from sporting activities, pain-free exercises, stretching exercises and non-steroidal anti-inflammatory drugs. Surgery may be necessary if these fail.

Reverse straight-leg raising test

Other name Femoral nerve tension test

Reverse straight-leg raising test is a maneuver which assesses femoral nerve tension. The patient lies in the prone position, the knee is flexed to 90° and, with the pelvis fixed to the table, the hip is extended. A positive test is one which reproduces anterior thigh radicular pain.

Rhabdomyolysis

Rhabdomyolysis (disintegration of striated muscle fibers with excretion of myoglobin in the urine) can occur after any very severe exertion (e.g. marathon running) and presents with muscle soreness. Recovery is usual, but renal failure can occur. Preventive measures include stretching exercises and warm up, and a gradual increase in training activities.

Rib fractures

Fractures of ribs can be due to a direct blow from, for example, a cricket ball or being crushed in a scrum. It can also occur spontaneously, as has occurred in novice golfers, probably due to excessive muscular action. The patient will complain of pain made worse by deep breathing. Fracture of the first rib may cause an audible snap and sudden shoulder pain made worse by deep breathing and movement of the arm. Pneumothorax can be a complication. Treatment involves pain relief using oral analgesics and a chest binder.

Rib stress fracture

Rib stress fractures can occur in rowers (possibly following a change from bow side to stroke side, or the reverse), canoeists and golfers. Fractures of the first rib also happen in baseball and basketball players. The clinical feature is an acute, sudden pain in the chest.

Rider's strain
See Adductor longus tendonitis

Rock climbers hand injuries

Rock climbers can develop hand injuries as a result of putting stresses on their fingers. They are likely to complain of stiffness in the fingers and aching in cold weather. Osteoarthritic changes can include contracture of proximal interphalangeal joints, osteophytes and subchondral cysts.

Rotator cuff disorders

Rotator cuff disorders can be due to overhead actions by baseball pitchers, volleyball players, tennis players, javelin throwers, swimmers and golfers. They are usually the result of repeated minor traumas, which can in time cause edema, hemorrhage, fibrosis, tendonitis and, in older patients, degeneration. A partial tear can occur in the act of throwing; a full thickness tear is most likely to occur in athletes over 50 years of age. Primary impingement is due to narrowing of the subacromial space by edema or by bony encroachment from the coracoacromial arch. Clinical features are pain, weakness, stiffness, impaired function and instability of the shoulder. The pain of impingement can occur at night and during complete rest. Physical findings are tenderness, a discrepancy between active and passive movements, and evidence of shoulder instability. Preventive measures include strengthening the shoulder muscles, generalized body conditioning and a good warm up. Conservative treatment involves strengthening and stretching exercises, reduction of activity, avoidance of overhead movements, ice, non-steroidal anti-inflammatory drugs and ultrasound. Surgery may be necessary if these measures fail.

Roux's sign

Roux's sign is a decrease in the distance between the greater trochanter and the pubis on the affected side of a fractured pelvis.

Rowe's sign

Rowe's sign is limitation in external rotation of the shoulder and restricted supination with the arm flexed forwards in chronic dislocation of the shoulder.

Rower's back injury

Rower's back injury is slipping of the intervertebral disc with pain in the buttock and leg. It is more likely to occur during weight-lifting training than in rowing. Precipitating factors can be excessive training, lack of warm-up exercises, prolonged endurance trials and the use of big rowing blades ('cleavers').

Runner's knee

See Iliotibial band friction syndrome

Runner's trots

Runner's trots is a gastrointestinal disorder liable to occur in long-distance runners, in training and in a race. Clinical features are abdominal cramp, bloating, frequent watery stools and sometimes melena.

S

Sacroiliac strain

Sacroiliac strain is due to stretching and tearing of the ligaments supporting the sacroiliac joint. Clinical features are pain around the join radiating to the groin, thigh and lower part of the back. This is reproduced by straight leg raising, forward flexion of the trunk with knees extended and Gaenslen's test. Treatment involves rest, analgesics and heat.

Saphenous nerve entrapment

The saphenous nerve can be entrapped by the fasciae of the vastus medialis, sartorius and adductor longus muscles as it emerges from the adductor canal. Clinical features are pain in the medial aspect of the knee, tenderness over the adductor canal and sensory changes in the sensory distribution of the nerve. The pain is made worse by walking, running and jumping. Treatment involves either rest, ice and anti-inflammatory drugs, or saphenous nerve block with bupivacaine and corticosteroid. If these fail, surgical release of the nerve at the point of entrapment is necessary.

Scalp laceration

Scalp laceration can occur in footballers, skiers, ice hockey players and riders. Treatment involves a thorough cleaning of the wound to remove all dirt, rinsing with plain water and covering with a sterile dressing. Deep lacerations may require stitching.

Scaphocapitate syndrome

Scaphocapitate syndrome is a fracture of the scaphoid bone associated with trans-scaphoid–transcapitate, perilunate fracture-dislocation, which causes a major disarrangement of the anatomy of the wrist. Surgical treatment may be necessary.

Scaphoid fracture

Fracture of the scaphoid bone is the most common fracture of the carpus. It is likely to occur in footballers, gymnasts and contact sports players, and is due to falling onto a hyperextended wrist. Clinical features are pain, tenderness and swelling in the 'anatomical snuffbox'. Treatment of a non-displaced fracture is a minimum of 6 weeks in a thumb spica casting. A displaced fracture requires open reduction and long-term immobilization for about 3 months. Non-union, malunion and avascular necrosis can be complications even with adequate treatment. In the long term arthritis can develop.

Scapholunate instability

Scapholunate instability can be acute or chronic. Acute instability follows a blow or fall with the wrist hyperextended. Clinical features are pain, tenderness and swelling over the joint. Chronic instability is a persistence of pain and disability for 3 months or more, by which time degenerative changes may have occurred in the joint. X-ray of an acute injury is likely to show widening of the scapholunate interval of more than 2 mm, a shortened appearance of the scaphoid bone and a scapholunate angle of more than 70°. Treatment for an acute injury can involve cast immobilization or surgery, but for chronic injury it is scapholunate arthrodesis.

Scapular fractures

Scapular fractures can be fracture of the body, the coracoid process, the glenoid neck, the acromion and the spine. They are usually the result of severe trauma, such as falling off a motorcycle or in football, hockey or a rugby scrum. There is likely to be an associated fracture of the spine, sternum and ribs, with shoulder girdle dislocation, brachial plexus injury, pneumothorax or emphysema. The patient complains of pain and presents with his arm adducted and protected from movement.

Fracture of the body is the most common fracture and is commonly associated with other injuries. Treatment involves support and ice.

Fracture of the coracoid process is uncommon and can be associated with acromioclavicular injury. It can be a stress fracture. The patient complains of pain, which may be localized to the front of the shoulder, and there is likely to be localized tenderness. Treatment is conservative, but surgery may be required for non-union.

Fracture of the glenoid neck is the second most common fracture and may be impacted. Treatment may involve closed treatment or open reduction.

Fracture of the acromion is rare. It can be due to a downward blow and there may be an associated brachial plexus injury. Displacement is usually slight, so most can be treated conservatively.

Fracture of the spine is usually associated with a fracture of the body and requires conservative treatment.

Scapulocostal syndrome
See Levator scapulae syndrome

Scapulothoracic bursitis
See Levator scapulae syndrome

Sciatic nerve contusion

Sciatic nerve contusion is due to a blow to the buttock and is characterized by pain in the buttock, back of thigh, foot and, sometimes, the whole sensory distribution of the nerve. Treatment involves analgesics and rest.

Scoring systems

Scoring systems of injuries are designed to provide an accurate audit of patient data, to define the extent of disability and functional recovery, and to evaluate health care. Scoring systems can be either anatomical, physiological or anatomical and physiological.

Anatomical scoring systems. The Abbreviated Injury Scale (AIS) is anatomically based and divides the body into regions, with each region being assigned a severity rating score of between one and six; this represents a sliding scale from minor to unsurvivable. It was revised (AIS-95) to include penetrating injuries. The alternative Injury Severity Score (ISS), which is based on AIS, divides the body into six regions and assesses the overall severity of multiple injuries.

Physiological scoring systems. The Glasgow Coma Scale and the Glasgow Coma Scale for Children (I and II) are used to assess brain damage. The Triage Index (TI) is an assessment of injury severity which measures dysfunction in the central nervous, cardiovascular and respiratory systems. The Trauma Score (TS) and the

Revised Trauma Score (RTS) are modifications of this index. The Acute Physiology and Chronic Health Evaluation (APACHE), with its modifications APACHE I and APACHE II, aim at predicting the severity of the injury, the prognosis and the degree of nursing care required. Finally, the Respiratory Index (RI) measures the patient's respiratory status.

Combined anatomical and physiological systems. The Injury Severity Score (ISS) and the Revised Trauma Score (RTS) are combined in the Trauma Revised Injury Severity Score (TRISS). A Severity Characterization of Trauma (ASCOT) is another combined system, as is the Pediatric Trauma Score (PTS) which has been designed specially for children.

See also Glasgow Coma Scale, Glasgow Coma Scale for Children

Scuba diver's decompression sickness

Decompression during scuba diving can cause fatigue, malaise, headache, disturbances of consciousness, mood, speech and co-ordination, sensory and motor nerve disturbances, girdle pain, sphincter control loss, joint pain, dyspnea, cough, chest pain, hemoptysis, cyanosis, pneumothorax, enlarged lymph nodes and lymphedema. Treatment involves the administration of oxygen and hydration followed by removal to a special treatment unit.

See also Decompression sickness

Second impact syndrome

Second impact syndrome is due to a blow to the head in a contact sport when the patient is still showing some symptoms of concussion or post-concussion due to a previous blow. Brain swelling is made worse and there is likely to be a further deterioration in the patient's physical and mental state, a deterioration which may become permanent.

Semimembranosus insertional tendonitis

Semimembranosus insertional tendonitis can occur in runners, jumpers and basketball and volleyball players. It presents with acute pain at the insertion of the tendon into the tibia. It can become chronic. Treatment involves rest, ice, non-steroidal anti-inflammatory drugs and wearing a knee support. Surgery may be required if the conservative measures fail.

Sesamoid chondromalacia

See Sesamoiditis

Sesamoid fracture

The two sesamoid bones in the tendons of flexor hallucis brevis can be fractured in footballers; synovitis of the metatarsophalangeal joint may be present. Clinical features are pain, swelling and restriction of movement. Stress fracture of the bone can occur in long-distance runners and footballers as an isolated lesion or as a feature of a plantar hyperextension injury ('turf toe') and causes a chronic impact and push-off disability. Treatment involves rest, non-steroidal anti-inflammatory drugs and taping the great toe in a neutral position. Surgery is required for non-union.

Sesamoiditis

Other name Sesamoid chondromalacia

Sesamoiditis is pain, tenderness and inflammation in the foot due to lesions of the two sesamoid bones in the tendons of flexor hallucis. The lesion may be a stress fracture, a fracture or a degeneration resembling chondromalacia of the patella. It is most common in young athletes and is made worse by running, jogging and weight bearing. Treatment is conservative, involving support with a sponge rubber pad and a corticosteroid injection. Surgical excision of the sesamoids may be needed.

Sever's disease

Other name Calcaneal apophysitis

Sever's disease is heel pain in child athletes aged between 5 and 12 years. It is due to calcaneal apophysitis and abnormalities of an apophysis, and can occur in both heels. Prevention is by wearing the appropriate shoes. Treatment involves wearing heel cups or pads, using non-steroidal anti-inflammatory drugs and performing exercises to strengthen the leg and ankle dorsiflexion. Athletic activities can be resumed when symptoms have subsided.

Shallow water blackout

Shallow water blackout is a temporary loss of consciousness of a diver who is breathing pure oxygen in shallow water. It may be due to a lowering of the syncope threshold or to the vasoconstrictive action of oxygen.

Shin-splints

See Medial tibial stress syndrome

Short-leg syndrome

Short-leg syndrome can occur in runners who are running on a cambered road or a banked surface. An abnormal stress is put on one side of the body, with increasing secondary pronation on the inner leg which can lead to trochanteric bursitis or iliotibial band friction syndrome.

Shoulder impingement syndrome

Shoulder impingement syndrome is due to an impingement of the soft tissues in the subacromial space and loss of the normal gliding mechanisms of the shoulder joint. Risk factors are a prominent anterior acromion and bony spurs arising from the acromioclavicular joint and under the acromion. It is liable to occur in athletes who engage in repeated overhead activity of the arm as in tennis, throwing and swimming. Clinical features include edema and inflammation of the supraspinatus tendon which are followed by degeneration or rupture of the tendon. The patient complains of weakness, stiffness and pain in the shoulder. On abduction of the arm from the side there is painless movement through the first 70–80° of abduction, then painful movement up to 120°, followed by further painless movement. Treatment can be conservative, involving rest of the shoulder, non-steroidal anti-inflammatory drugs to reduce pain and inflammation, infiltration of the subacromial space by local anesthetic (2–3 ml) and corticosteroid (1 ml), physical therapy using ice, heat or ultrasound, and mobilization. Surgery may be recommended for recurrent or chronic pain which does not respond to conservative treatment, and for biceps tendon involvement and cuff tears.

Shoulder joint dislocation

See Shoulder joint subluxation and dislocation

Shoulder joint instability

Shoulder joint instability can occur in swimmers. The joint is inherently unstable, and during a swimming stroke a partial dislocation of the head of the humerus can injure the glenoid labrum and cause an impingement syndrome.

See also Impingement syndrome

Shoulder joint subluxation and dislocation

Other name Glenohumeral subluxation and dislocation

Instability of the shoulder joint can lead to subluxation and dislocation. Subluxation is an increase in the translation of the head of the humerus on the glenoid cavity of the scapula without complete dislocation. Factors contributing to the instability of the joint are laxness of the capsule and its ligaments, dysfunction and lack of synchrony and co-ordination of muscles acting on the joint, a bony defect of the glenoid rim, detachment of the glenoid labrum with disruption of the anterior capsule, a congenitally small labrum and a bony defect of the head of the humerus. Ligamentous laxity may be present in other joints. Subluxations and dislocations can occur in throwing sports, football, swimming, tennis and badminton. They can be acute, recurrent and chronic (locked). They can also be anterior, posterior or multidirectional.

Anterior subluxation can be due to a sudden effort or to multiple microtrauma. The patient complains of pain (which may be localized posteriorly), clicking and impairment of movement in some activities. Dead arm syndrome can be a feature and rotator cuff impingement symptoms are common. Treatment involves non-steroidal anti-inflammatory drugs, immobilization of the arm in a sling for 4–5 weeks and rehabilitation exercises.

Anterior dislocation is the most common of the shoulder dislocations, accounting for over 90% of cases overall. The head of the humerus is usually dislocated into the subcoracoid position. The axillary nerve may be damaged, but there is little or no damage to soft tissue. The patient complains of pain and presents with the arm held slightly abducted and externally rotated; internal rotation and full abduction are impossible. The head of the humerus may be palpable. Treatment involves reduction as soon as possible and before muscle spasm begins. Recurrence is common in young patients, especially in men, with the patient complaining of the shoulder popping out, and they may be able to produce it voluntarily.

Posterior subluxation is less common than anterior subluxation, but more common than posterior dislocation. It is usually due to multiple microtrauma and not to a single event. The patient presents with shoulder pain, which is made worse when the arm is flexed, adducted and internally rotated. Treatment involves immobilization and non-steroid anti-inflammatory drugs. It can be recurrent.

Posterior dislocation is much less common than anterior dislocation. It can be due to a fall on an outstretched hand or to a direct blow on the shoulder. The patient presents with the arm adducted and internally rotated. The coracoid process is prominent. Fracture of the lesser tuberosity of the humerus can be a complication. Recurrent and chronic dislocation can sometimes occur. Treatment involves conservative measures and, if these fail, surgery.

Multidirectional instability is instability occurring in more than one plane, with anterior–inferior being the most common direction due to the presence of a large inferior capsular pouch. It may be bilateral and about 50% of patients have general joint laxity.

See also Dead arm syndrome, rotator cuff syndrome

Sindig–Larsen–Johannson syndrome

Other name Patellar osteochondritis dissecans

Sindig–Larsen–Johannson syndrome is a chronic traction injury of the lower pole (rarely the upper pole) of the patella. It is most common in boys aged 10–15 years and is caused, and made worse, by running and jumping. It can be bilateral. Clinical features are likely to be pain at the pole, pain when pressure is applied to patellofemoral joint, crepitus and effusion into the joint.

Sinus tarsi syndrome

Sinus tarsi syndrome follows a sprain to the ankle. Clinical features are pain and tenderness of the lateral opening of the sinus tarsi (the space between the calcaneus and the talus) and a feeling of instability in the hind foot when walking over uneven ground. The pain can be severe when standing, walking on even ground and during supination and adduction of the foot; the pain usually disappears with rest.

Ski-boot neuropathy

Ski-boot neuropathy is rupture of the extensor hallucis longus tendon associated with sensory nerve dysfunction in the skin of the dorsum of the foot due to pressure and friction from a ski-boot.

Ski-boot-top fracture

Ski-boot-top fracture is a fracture of the tibia in young skiers who fall forwards. It occurs at the level of the fulcrum of the top of the boot, at the upper margin of the inner lining, 2–5 cm above the ankle joint.

Skier's thumb

Skier's thumb is a sprain of the ulnar collateral ligament of the thumb following a fall forward onto an outstretched hand with the pole forcing the thumb into abduction and hyperextension. Clinical features are a painful and swollen thumb. A tear of the ligament may be partial or complete. A partial tear is treated conservatively; a complete tear may be treated conservatively or by surgery.

Ski-pole thumb injury

Ski-pole thumb injury is a tear of the ulnar collateral ligament of the metacarpophalangeal joint of the thumb. It is due to a combined extension and radially deviating stress when a skier falls on an outstretched hand and his or her thumb is jammed against the ski pole. Avulsion of the collateral ligament from the base of the proximal phalanx, with or without a fragment of bone being torn off, is associated with tearing of the palmar plate and accessory collateral ligament. In a Stener lesion the aponeurosis is interposed between the two ends of the torn ligament, which prevents healing.

Snapping hip syndrome

Snapping hip syndrome is a loud slapping noise over the lateral aspect of the thigh produced by movements of the hip in athletes and ballet dancers. The most common cause is slipping of the iliotibial band over the greater tuberosity of the femur; it can produce trochanteric bursitis. Other causes are slipping of the long head of biceps femoris over the ischial tuberosity, slipping of the iliofemoral ligaments over the femoral head, slipping of the iliopsoas tendon over the iliopectineal eminence and loose bodies in the hip joint. The patient should be reassured of the benign nature of the condition and could try to limit movements liable to cause the snapping.

Sollerman's test

Sollerman's test assesses hand function while a patient carries out 20 activity-of-daily-living tasks in which all the types of hand grip are used. The speed at which the tests are carried out is timed.

Speed's test

Speed's test is used in the evaluation of a rotator cuff disorder. It is carried out by resisted forward elevation of the humerus against an extended elbow. Pain is produced if the biceps tendon is involved in the disorder.

Spondylolisthesis

Spondylolisthesis is the forward displacement of one vertebra over the vertebra below it; it usually occurs at L4–5, but it can occur at a higher level. It is a result of repetitive hyperextension of the lumbar spine which can lead eventually to a stress fracture and spondylosis (a defect in the interarticular area). Clinical features are low back pain and muscle spasm. Treatment involves stopping all hyperextensive movements and other sporting activities, and wearing a lumbosacral orthosis (this is worn for as long as there is pain, which can be 6 months). A rehabilitation program is then necessary. Surgical treatment may be required for severe cases which have not responded to treatment and where there is nerve root entrapment and intractable root pain.

Spondylolysis

Spondylolysis is a defect of the pars interarticularis which allows one vertebral body to slip forward over another. It is occasionally due to a congenital abnormality, but it is usually due to repeated stresses. It can present in adolescence or later in life. Athletes likely to present with it are gymnasts, American football players, baseball players, weight-lifters, rowers, wrestlers and tennis players. Clinical features are a chronic low back pain which may be unilateral and involve the buttocks and posterior thighs, lordosis, hamstring tightness and weak abdominal muscles. A tennis player will complain of the pain when serving. Active or passive extension of the spine and standing on one leg produces or increases the pain. X-ray of the spine confirms the diagnosis. Treatment can involve bed rest to relieve the pain, a restriction of activities and the wearing a rigid lumbosacral brace in combination with exercises to strengthen the abdominal muscles and stretch the lumbodorsal fascia.

Sprinter's fracture

Sprinter's fracture is an avulsion of the origins of the hamstring muscles from the ischial tuberosity which can occur when a sprinter is starting from a block or increasing speed. He or she may fall over. Treatment involves rest for several weeks.

Squeeze test

The squeeze test assesses whether tibiofibular syndesmosis is present. The leg is squeezed by the examiner's hand just above the midpoint of the calf. The test is positive when proximal compression produces distal pain in the area of the interosseous membrane or its supporting structures.

Sternoclavicular joint injury

Sternoclavicular joint injury can be either a ligamentous sprain, subluxation of the joint with partial ligamentous and capsular disruption, or dislocation anteriorly or posteriorly with complete ligamentous and capsular disruption. Dislocation of the joint is rare. The patient complains of pain in the joint which is made worse by any movement of the shoulder girdle. A posterior dislocation may be associated with pulmonary or vascular injury for which the patient must be examined. Treatment will depend on the type of injury. For a sprain it involves ice and support with a figure-of-eight bandage. An anterior dislocation will require reduction (which may have to be repeated as the reduction can be unstable) and support. Posterior dislocation needs reduction which may have to be open.

Stingers

Stingers is the popular name given by wrestlers for the effects of stretching the nerves in the brachial plexus or its nerve roots. Clinical features are severe electric shock-like pains in the arm, followed by a dull ache, weakness and numbness of the arm. The wrestler presents with the arm either hanging at the side or shaking the wrist and with impairment of muscle movement; the arm is likely to return to normal in about 5 minutes. If recovery does not take place within that time, treatment is necessary and involves the use of ice, non-steroidal anti-inflammatory drugs, transcutaneous electrical nerve stimulation and wearing a hard cervical collar. Recurrence is likely if the wrestler returns to the sport before full recovery. Permanent weakness and muscle atrophy can occur.

Straight-leg raising test

The straight-leg raising test assesses sciatic nerve root tension. With the patient lying supine, the leg is raised in full extension. A positive test is the production of pain in the leg before it is raised to 30–35°. Pain in the back is not a positive result.

Strain
See Muscle strain

Stress fracture

Stress fracture is a fracture of bone when it is subjected to repeated loading, the loading being less than that which causes an acute fracture. They can occur in novices and trained athletes. The fact that they are much more common in women than men has been attributed to women having thinner bones, but there is also an association with amenorrhea, menstruation irregularity and eating disorders. Other factors are the intensity of sport activity, bone mineralization, muscle fatigue and, possibly, hormonal variations. They are uncommon in children. Clinical features are usually a dull pain, tenderness and swelling at the site. Any stress fracture which extends into subchondral bone and articular cartilage is a risk factor for osteoarthritis.

See also Femoral neck fracture, femoral shaft stress fracture, fibular and tibial stress fracture, fifth metatarsal stress fracture, medial malleolar stress fracture, metatarsal stress fracture, navicular stress fracture, pubic bone stress fracture

S–T segment depression

Depression of the S–T segment may be found in an electrocardiogram (ECG) during exercise stress training. Older athletes require further investigation as the S–T segment depression can be diagnostic of myocardial ischemia. However, in a young athlete who is a non-smoker with normal blood pressure and serum cholesterol and who has a good exercise tolerance, the depression is not important.

Subastragalar dislocation

See Peritalar dislocation

Subchondral hematoma of the ear

Other name Cauliflower ear

Subchondral hematoma of the ear is a common boxing injury. If it is not drained, chondritis, loss of cartilage and a thickened and distorted ear are likely.

Subclavian vein thrombosis

See Effort thrombosis

Subcoracoid bursitis

Subcoracoid bursitis can occur in table-tennis players as a result of repeated medial rotation of the shoulder. Clinical features are pain localized to the anterior aspect of the shoulder and distal to the coracoid process of the scapula, pain produced by passive horizontal flexion of the arm across the chest, and an area of tenderness just below the tip of the coracoid process. Treatment can involve corticosteroid injection into the tender area.

Subdural hematoma

Subdural hematoma can be due to a contrecoup or a rotational acceleration–deceleration of the brain. It can be (a) blood in the subdural space without contusion of the surface of the brain or edema of the brain; or (b) blood in the subdural space with an underlying cerebral contusion and edema. The mortality for the first of these is about 20% and for the second more than 50%. Bridging veins between the brain and the cavernous sinus are torn and the hematoma develops slowly. Unconsciousness develops gradually with the slowly increasing intracranial pressure and may not be fully developed for hours or days.

Subtalar dislocation

See Peritalar dislocation

Subtalar instability and sprain

Subtalar instability (of the talonavicular and talocalcaneal joints) and sprain is usually associated with injury of the lateral ligament of the ankle. It is liable to occur while playing tennis, soccer, volleyball, squash and basketball. The patient complains that the ankle has given way and of stiffness, pain and swelling. Treatment involves rest, ice and immobilization.

Subungual exostosis

Subungual exostosis is a bony outgrowth on the dorsal surface of the terminal phalanx in the big toe (and occasionally other toes). It is a common condition in athletes. The patient complains of discomfort on running, jogging and long-distance walking. Pressure on the nail is tender. Diagnosis is made by X-ray. Treatment involves surgical excision.

Sudden death in athletes

Sudden death in athletes is uncommon, but occurs more frequently in athletes over 40 years of age than in younger athletes and is most likely to be due to unsuspected or mild cardiac disease. In child athletes death can be due to either a congenital malformation of the heart or coronary arteries, a viral infection or can follow an attack of rheumatic fever; boys under 14 years have been killed by a blow on the chest over the heart by a baseball. In older athletes the most common causes of death are:

(a) Coronary artery disease;

(b) Hypertrophic myocardiopathy;

(c) Right ventricular cardiomyopathy;

(d) Myocarditis;

(e) Idiopathic long Q–T interval;

(f) Marfan's syndrome; and

(g) Rupture of berry aneurysm.

See also Aortic rupture

Superficial peroneal nerve entrapment

Superficial peroneal nerve entrapment can occur at the exit of the nerve through an edge of fascia in the anterolateral aspect of the leg. It causes tingling and numbness in the dorsal aspect of the ankle and foot, except in the first web space (this is supplied by the deep peroneal nerve). The nerve is tender to percussion as it emerges from beneath the fascia. Treatment is surgical.

Superficial radial nerve compression

Superficial radial nerve compression is decreased sensation or numbness in the dorsal radial region of the hand and the dorsum of the thumb and index finger. It can occur in weight-lifters who are wearing a wrist band, a wrist watch or a leather support. Treatment involves rest, splinting and not wearing a wrist constrictor.

Superior scapular syndrome

See Levator scapulae syndrome

Suprascapular neuropathy

Suprascapular neuropathy can occur in volleyball players. Clinical features are a dull shoulder pain and weakness in abduction and external rotation of the arm due to denervation of the supraspinatus and infraspinatus muscles. This is followed by atrophy of the muscles. There may be no functional disability while playing volleyball.

Supraspinatus tendonitis

Supraspinatus tendonitis is a result of degeneration of the supraspinatus tendon as a result of hyaline degeneration of its collagen fibres. Clinical features are (a) pain over the shoulder on active or passive abduction (most commonly in the middle range of movement); (b) pain on bringing the arm down to the side, with the patient allowing the arm to drop past the painful area; and (c) a possible disturbance of the scapulohumeral rhythm during abduction. The greater tuberosity of the humerus may show pitting or sclerosis on a radiograph. There can be remission and aggravation of the pain over years. Management involves nonsteroidal anti-inflammatory drugs, local infiltration with a local anesthetic and corticosteroid (this is repeated if necessary at intervals for up to 4 weeks), and passive movement techniques. Surgery may be indicated if the condition becomes chronic or recurs frequently.

Supraspinatus tendon rupture

Supraspinatus tendon rupture can follow degeneration of the tendon and may be either incomplete or complete.

Incomplete rupture can occur in sportspeople as an acute injury with symptoms similar to those of supraspinatus tendonitis. Treatment is conservative.

Complete rupture can be acute or chronic, with the rupture occurring in the 'critical zone', an area just proximal to the insertion where the blood supply is relatively poor. Sometimes the tendon is avulsed from its insertion. The patient complains of feeling or hearing a snap in the shoulder and loss of strength and mobility in it. Active abduction of the shoulder is limited to about 20° and is accompanied by movement of the scapula and upwards shrugging of the shoulder. A gap in the tendon may be felt by palpating between the greater tuberosity and the acromion. A communication can develop between the subacromial bursa and the glenohumeral joint, and this can be demonstrated by ultra-sound or double-contrast arthrography. Surgical treatment involves decompression and direct repair, which can use part of the biceps tendon as a graft.

Sural nerve entrapment

Entrapment of the sural nerve, which can be due to the forma-tion of fibrous tissue around it following an injury to the back of the heel. This can cause numbness or pain in the lateral border of the foot, the fifth toe and, sometimes, the lateral half of the fourth toe. Percussion of the nerve behind the lateral malleolus can cause tingling. A neuroma may develop. Treatment can be either conservative by padding the shoe and steroid injection, or surgical when a neuroma has developed.

Swimmer's chlorine keratitis

Chlorine keratitis can occur in swimmers due to exposure of the cornea to chlorinated water which may lead to the loss of its superficial cells. The swimmer complains of pain and a sensation of something in the eye. Symptoms usually resolve in 1–2 days. Wearing goggles is a preventive measure.

Swimmer's conjunctivitis

Conjunctivitis in swimmers can be due to chemical irritation by pool or salt water. Wearing goggles reduces the incidence. Treatment involves the use of ophthalmic irrigation solutions.

Swimmer's corneal edema

Swimmer's corneal edema is a result of prolonged exposure of the eye to water. Edema of the cornea can cause halos due to abnormal bending of light rays and sensitivity of the eye to light. Wearing goggles is a preventive measure.

Swimmer's ear

Swimmer's ear is an acute or chronic otitis externa occurring in swimmers and is due to an infection by staphylococci, *Pseudomonas*, *Escherichia coli* or *Enterobacter aerogenes*. Clinical features of acute otitis externa are pain and swelling of the ear; infection can spread to the middle ear and cause deafness.

Swimmer's exostosis

Exostosis of the external auditory canal is a benign tumor of bone which is likely to occur in a swimmer who frequently swims in cold water. It presents usually as two or three smooth sessile growths on opposing surfaces of the bony canal near the annulus. They may be symptomless, but can cause an infection in the canal from retention of debris. Prevention involves careful drying of the canal after swimming. Surgical removal may be necessary.

Swimmer's knee

Swimmer's knee is pain in the knee due to either (a) repeated stretching of the medial collateral ligament (rarely rupture of it) during the breaststroke kick; (b) instability and dislocation of the patella; or (c) chondromalacia (softening of the articular cartilage). The test for instability is the apprehension test, which is positive when the patient has a sensation of instability when the patella is pushed laterally. With chondromalacia of the knee there is grating at the patellofemoral joint, tenderness when the patella is compressed against the femur and pain in front of the knee which is exacerbated by activity but relieved by holding the knee in extension. Effusion into the knee is minimal or absent. Treatment of swimmer's knee involves rest, ice, non-steroidal anti-inflammatory drugs, strengthening of vastus medialis and a knee brace to prevent lateral patellar tracking.

Swimmer's shoulder

Swimmer's shoulder is a condition similar to impingement syndrome. It is likely to occur in older swimmers with partial or complete rotator cuff tears. It is due to strain being put upon biceps and supraspinatus tendons in butterfly and freestyle strokes. Treatment involves changes in the training program; the type of stroke may have to be altered. If the condition has not improved in 12 months, division of the coracoacromial ligament may be necessary.

Swimming pool granuloma

Other name Mycobacterium marinum infection

Swimming pool granuloma is due to infection by *Mycobacterium marinum,* a micro-organism which inhabits fresh and salt-water and can cause disease in fish. Swimmers can be infected through skin lesions, with the production of a granulomatous patch which ulcerates in an immunocompromised patient to form an ulcer with undermined edges and a necrotic base. Tendon sheaths and synovia can be invaded. Minor lesions heal spontaneously.

T

Tailor's bunion
See Bunionette

Talar tilt test
See Inversion stress test

Talotibial exostoses

Talotibial exostoses are bony outgrowths around the ankle joint and on the surface of the talus. They can be a complication of athlete's ankle (anterior tibiotalar impingement) and the result of localized cyclic overloading of bone with the production of microfractures. They are particularly common in ballet dancers. The athlete complains of pain in the ankle, especially on running or going downstairs, of a loss of speed when pushing off to run and of a dull ache at other times. On examination there is tenderness over the neck of the talus or the anterior border of the tibia at the joint and restricted and painful extension of the ankle, sometimes with a palpable exostosis. An exostosis may break off, become a loose foreign body within the joint and cause locking of the joint. Osteoarthritis is a complication. The diagnosis is confirmed by X-ray. Although treatment can be conservative, involving rest, non-steroidal anti-inflammatory drugs and injection of corticosteroid and local anesthetic, surgical exostectomy is necessary to cure the condition.

See also Athlete's ankle

Talus lateral process stress fracture

Talus lateral process stress fracture can be due to repetitive loading. Clinical features are pain in the posterior ankle joint, pain on walking and restriction in mobility of the subtalar joint.

Primary radiographic findings are minimal or misleading. Treatment is conservative.

Tarsal navicular stress fracture

Tarsal navicular stress fracture can occur in runners and jumpers. Clinical features are a dull pain and tenderness in the medial arch region. The fracture can be partial. Treatment involves immobilization in plaster for 6–8 weeks.

Tarsal tunnel syndrome

Tarsal tunnel syndrome is due to compression of the posterior tibial nerve in the tarsal tunnel by a space-occupying lesion. It is characterized by paresthesiae and pain in the area of the foot supplied by posterior tibial nerve. Although involving treatment can be conservative by immobilization, non-steroidal anti-inflammatory drugs and injection of a steroid preparation, surgical decompression of the tunnel is usually required.

Tarsometatarsal dislocation and fracture-dislocation

Tarsometatarsal dislocation and fracture-dislocation are rare injuries which can occur in severe trauma to the foot. They also occur in American football. Clinical features are pain and swelling. The diagnosis is confirmed by X-ray. Treatment involves reduction which may be closed or open. Complications are vascular damage which can cause ischemia of the forefoot and gangrene of the toes, ankylosis and osteoarthritis.

Tendinosis

Tendinosis is a degenerative condition of tendons in which there are areas of local necrosis without an inflammatory response. It is asymptomatic, but is a cause of spontaneous rupture of tendons.

Tennis elbow

Tennis elbow is epicondylitis, lateral or medial. Although it is described as occurring in tennis players, it is more likely to be associated with other sports in which the arms are used intensely (e.g. gymnastics, baseball, badminton and swimming) and it can occur in people who have never played tennis. It occurs most commonly in the fourth decade. The pathological causes are uncertain; however, it has been attributed to chronic periostitis of the humeral condyles with spur formation, a partial tear of the common extensor tendon (or to granulation tissue in it), traumatic capsulitis of the radiohumeral joint, chondromalacia of the radial head and radioulnar bursitis.

Lateral epicondylitis is seven times more common than medial epicondylitis. The onset can be gradual or sudden. It presents with pain anterior and distal to the lateral epicondyle of the humerus. The pain is made worse by playing backhanded strokes in tennis, shaking hands and picking up a full cup. Pressure on the epicondyle produces little or no pain, but pressure over the origin of extensor carpi radialis brevis can cause severe pain.

Medial epicondylitis presents with pain at, or just distal to, the medial epicondyle on making either wrist flexion or forearm pronation movements. Pressure on the attachments points of pronator teres and flexor carpi radialis to the medial epicondyle causes severe pain.

In tennis players treatment can be non-operative, involving changes in technique, a change in the size of the racket handle and isotonic eccentric exercises. The tennis player should wear a tennis elbow-strap and learn to meet a backhand stroke in front. There are several surgical options, none of which is consistently satisfactory.

Tennis leg

Other name Gastrocnemius tear

Tennis leg is due to a tear of the medial head of the gastrocnemius muscle at its musculotendinous junction. It is most likely to occur in middle-aged people playing tennis or engaged in other athletic activities. It presents as a sudden severe pain in the calf, making the patient believe that he or she has been hit with a stick or stone. With a slight tear the patient can limp in pain on his or her toes, but with a large tear walking is impossible. Pain in the calf can be reproduced by dorsiflexing the ankle. The belly of gastrocnemius may be swollen, with bruising at the site of the tear, and pressure on calf veins can sometimes cause a deep venous thrombosis. Treatment involves rest with the leg elevated, ice applied to the spot, an elastic stocking, graduated exercises and walking at first with a crutch and then with a stick.

Tennis toe

Tennis toe is a subungual hemorrhage under the nail plate of the big toe. It can be very painful and immediate evacuation of the blood is necessary.

Tenoperiostitis

Tenoperiostitis is an overuse injury affecting the insertion of a tendon into a bone with inflammation due to repeated stress at the periosteal attachment. It is most common at the elbow (e.g. tennis elbow and golfer's elbow), at the attachment of adductor longus, at the proximal and distal attachments of the patellar tendon, and at the insertion of Achilles tendon into the calcaneus. Clinical features are pain, tenderness and localized swelling at the site. Treatment involves rest, support, oral non-steroidal anti-inflammatory drugs and local steroid injection.

See also Golfer's elbow, tennis elbow

Tenpin-bowling hand syndrome

Tenpin-bowling hand syndrome is characterized by discomfort, dull pain, and attacks of sharp pain in the fourth and fifth fingers as well as the medial side of the hand due to the pressure and weight of the heavy bowl. There is an association with tennis elbow. Treatment involves a rest from bowling.

Terry Thomas sign

Terry Thomas sign is a widening of the space between the scaphoid bone and the lunate due to disruption of the intracarpal scapholunate ligament. It is named after an English comedian whose upper incisor teeth were widely spaced, which was obvious when he smiled or laughed.

Testicular trauma

Other name 'One-ball-left' syndrome

Testicular trauma is the result of a direct blow in which a testis is either driven against the pelvis or hit by a cricket ball or other hard ball that was travelling fast. The testis is ruptured, the tunica albuginea is torn, the seminiferous tubules are extruded into the tunica vaginalis, and a hematocele forms. Clinical features are very severe pain, a tender mass and fever. Complications are infection and atrophy of the testis. Treatment involves early exploration, which reduces the morbidity and increases the chance of saving the testis.

Thomas' elbow
See Little League elbow

Thoracic outlet syndrome

Thoracic outlet syndrome is due to compression of the subclavian artery, subclavian vein or brachial plexus as they pass between the clavicle in front and the first rib and anterior and posterior scalene muscles behind, and enter the axilla. Other factors that may play a part are a cervical rib, abnormal scalene muscles, adventitial fibrous bands and drooping of the shoulder in older athletes. It can occur in throwers, weight-lifters and footballers. Clinical features can be paresthesiae in the arm, a cold hand, vasospasm, venous congestion and claudication. Treatment is at first conservative but, if these are unsuccessful, thoracic outlet decompression is performed by either first rib resection or cervical rib removal.

Thoracic spine injuries

Thoracic spine injuries are uncommon in athletes, but they can occur in football and other contact sports.

Soft tissue injuries are sprains or contusions. The patient complains of pain and tenderness, with the pain localized to a small area. Muscle sprain can produce tenderness over a larger area. The presence of an underlying fracture can be suggested by the history of a severe direct blow and a localized area of tenderness. Immediate treatment involves cold therapy, such as ice applied to the site, and this is followed by reconditioning and rehabilitation.

Spinal contusion is usually due to a direct blow, such as from an American football helmet. The patient is likely to complain of pain, tenderness and a loss in the range of spinal movement. Treatment is similar to that for a soft tissue injury.

Compression fracture of the thoracic spine usually follows severe trauma in young athletes, but in older athletes with osteoporotic bone the force causing the injury may not be so great. The patient is likely to remember the trauma, complains of pain and adopts a kyphotic attitude to relieve it. Considerable paraspinal pain is present. X-ray shows the compression. The patient should be questioned about any transient paraplegia and examined for evidence of spinal cord injury. Treatment involves analgesics and immobilization by an orthotic device, which is in place for about 6 weeks in a young athlete and about 12 weeks in an older athlete with osteoporosis. This is followed by rehabilitation. Return to non-contact sports is then allowed, but the patient is warned against the risks of engaging in contact sports.

Transverse process fracture can occur in contact sports as the result of a direct blow from, for instance, an American football helmet. Pain is immediate and acute. There is tenderness over the fracture and to relieve pain the patient may adopt a scoliotic or kyphotic posture. The fracture is usually visible on a plain X-ray; if not, it can be identified by tomography. Associated features can be painful respiration and reduced breathing. Treatment involves cold therapy with ice, followed by massage, stretching and rehabilitation.

Thoracic fracture-dislocation can occur in high diving, sky diving and automobile racing accidents. It is usually associated with some degree of spinal cord injury, and the treatment given will depend on the degree of this injury. Recommended treatment for (a) a patient with an incomplete neurological deficit is spinal realignment, spinal cord decompression and internal fixation with fusion of the spine; and for (b) a patient with a complete neurological deficit is immobilization in a brace and rehabilitation.

Tibialis posterior syndrome

Tibialis posterior syndrome is a chronic tenosynovitis of the posterotibial tendon at the lower end of the tibia and behind the medial malleolus. It presents as pain, tenderness and swelling in the inner aspect of the shin and ankle. It occurs most frequently in flat-footed road runners.

Tibial proximal epiphysis fracture

Fracture of the proximal epiphysis of the tibia can occur in adolescent basketball and volleyball players before full skeletal maturity has been achieved. It can be due to either hyperextension of the knee following a jump or a strong contraction of quadriceps in deceleration. Clinical features are pain, swelling, inability to stand on the leg and inability to extend the knee actively. X-ray confirms the diagnosis. The fracture can be extra-articular (can be treated conservatively) or intra-articular (for which surgery is necessary).

Tibial stress fracture
See Fibular and tibial stress fracture

Tibiofibular proximal joint disorders

Disorders of the proximal tibiofibular joint can be subluxation or dislocation. Dislocation can be anterolateral, anteromedial or superior. These can result from a fall on an adducted leg with the knee in flexion and the foot in plantar flexion and inversion, as can occur during a slide tackle in soccer. The patient complains of pain and tenderness over the joint and there may be deficiency in full extension of the knee. In subluxation the instability is detected by pressure on the head of the fibula. The instability can become chronic, with discomfort and deficiency in full knee extension. Recurrence is common. Treatment of an acute injury is by closed reduction, an elastic bandage and the use of a crutch. Chronic instability may require surgery.

Tibiofibular synostosis

Tibiofibular synostosis is an area of bony union in the inter-osseous membrane which can be due to trauma or ankle sprains involving the interosseous membrane. Clinical features can be tenderness over the site, pain on weight bearing or movement of the ankle and limitation of dorsiflexion at the ankle. The condition may be symptomless. Treatment in the first place can be conservative, involving a reduction in activity and non-steroidal anti-inflammatory drugs. Surgical excision may be necessary, but should be postponed until the lesion is mature in order to prevent recurrence.

Tinea pedis
See Athlete's foot

Tinel's test

Tinel's test assesses whether carpal tunnel syndrome is present. The test is positive if a tingling or an electrical shock feeling is produced in the distribution of the median nerve when tapping proximally to, directly over and distally to the palmar wrist creases.

See also Carpal tunnel syndrome

Traumatic arthritis

Traumatic arthritis of the small joints of the hand can occur in golfers due to repeated striking of the ball. Clinical features are pain, tenderness and restricted movements. Treatment involves rest, non-steroidal anti-inflammatory drugs and playing with a specially designed grip of the club.

Traumatic hemorrhages of the skin

Traumatic hemorrhages of the skin can occur in fast bowlers in cricket and in players of tennis, basketball, squash and other games which involve rapid stops and starts. Hemorrhages into the skin can occur as 'black haloes' and splinter hemorrhages. If the very painful subungual hematoma occurs, immediate evacuation is required.

Trench foot

Trench foot derives its name from the condition affecting soldiers in trenches during the First World War. It is due to prolonged exposure of the feet to cold and wet conditions, with tight boots, fatigue and immobility being conributing factors. The feet are swollen, cold, white or purplish, and the patient may have difficulty in walking. Treatment involves removing the causative factors and allowing the feet to recover spontaneously. Recovery can be accompanied by severe pain. Complications can be permanent anesthesia, hyperesthesiae, ulceration of the skin and gangrene.

Triceps tendon rupture

Rupture of tendon of triceps can occur in weight-lifters or from a fall on to an outstretched arm. Clinical features are pain, bruising and swelling of the elbow posteriorly. The condition may, for a time, be unrecognized and present later with features similar to those of cubital tunnel syndrome. Treatment is surgical.

Triquetral fracture

Fracture of the triquetrum can be due to hyperextension of the wrist with impingement of the end of the ulna on the triquetrum. Clinical features are pain and tenderness over the fracture. Treatment involves immobilization for 3–4 weeks. Non-union can occur, but is not important.

Triquetrohamate and triquetrolunate instability

Triquetrohamate and triquetrolunate instability are forms of carpal instability. There may or may not have been a history of trauma. The patient may complain of an audible or palpable clink or clunk and there is tenderness over the joint. Treatment involves immobilization, non-steroidal anti-inflammatory drugs and corticosteroid injection into the joint. Surgery may be necessary if these methods are unsuccessful.

Trochanteric bursitis

Trochanteric bursitis can be due to a blow or to irritation by the iliotibial band. Clinical features are pain and tenderness. Treatment involves non-steroidal anti-inflammatory drugs and exercises to strengthen the gluteal muscles and to stretch the iliotibial band and fascia lata. If these measures fail, a corticosteroid can be injected locally.

Turf toe
See Metatarsophalangeal joint injuries

U

Ugly parent syndrome

Ugly parent syndrome is a term used in sports medicine to describe the adverse effects on a young sportsperson or athlete caused by the ambitious parent seeking to obtain self-gratification from the success of the child and coercing the child into excessive training, applying massive pressure from the sideline during a competition, and often inciting violence during contact sports. Success causes the parent to preen himself or herself; failure induces feelings of anger and frustration.

Ulnar nerve compression in the canal of Guyon

The canal of Guyon in the wrist is radial to the pisiform bone, ulnar to the hook of the hamate bone, roofed by the superficial part of the flexor retinaculum, and floored by the flexor retinaculum and the pisohamate ligament; it contains the ulnar nerve and ulnar artery. Compression of the ulnar nerve in the canal can occur in a cyclist with poorly padded handlebars and an incorrect placement of the hands on the bars. Clinical features are numbness, paresthesiae and pain in the part of the hands supplied by the nerve. Management involves improving technique, having good padding on the bicycle's handlebars or wearing padded gloves.

See also Hypothenar hammer syndrome

Ulnar neuritis

Ulnar neuritis can occur in throwers, baseball pitchers and cross-country skiers. It can be due to (a) hypermobility of the ulnar nerve which can sublux out of the tunnel on the back of the medial humeral epicondyle during rapid flexion and extension of the elbow; (b) traction on the nerve from valgus instability; and (c) cubital irritation. Clinical features can be numbness of the fifth finger and of the ulnar half of the fourth finger, medial elbow aching and weakness of the hand in throwing.

V

Valgus overload

Valgus overload is a condition which can occur in baseball pitchers and javelin throwers. They complain of pain over the olecranon medially and posteriorly. There is also loss in control while throwing due to the excessive valgus stress which is applied to the elbow, driving the olecranon into the olecranon fossa; a cartilaginous or bony osteophyte may be present. Treatment involves physiotherapy; surgery is necessary if an osteophyte is present.

Verrucae
See Warts

Vibrio parahaemolyticus infection

Vibrio parahaemolyticus is a curved motile Gram-negative bacillus which is present in coastal and estuarine waters. It can cause septicemia in swimmers and water-skiers with an abrasion or open wound through which the organism can enter the body.

Warts

Other name Verrucae

Warts are due to infection by the human papilloma virus (HPV), which causes benign, spontaneously regressing tumors of the skin, especially on the hands and feet. They are particularly liable to occur on users of sport centers, gymnasiums and swimming pools. They can be single or multiple. A deep endophytic type on the foot is caused by HPV-1 and can be extremely painful. A mosaic-like type caused by HPV-2 is usually shallow and painless. Regression generally occurs in 6–8 months.

Water polo injuries

Water polo injuries are due mainly to throwing the ball and are the same as those produced in other throwing sports and in swimming. They are likely to be impingement syndrome, rotator cuff tendonitis, acromioclavicular joint degeneration, shoulder dislocation and medial epicondylitis at the elbow.

Watson's test

Watson's test is a maneuver to assess scapholunate instability. The examiner stabilizes the volar aspect of the scaphoid with the wrist held in ulnar deviation and the patient's hand is then brought from ulnar into radial deviation. The test is positive when pain is produced by the injured scapholunate ligaments.

Weight-lifter's shoulder

Weight-lifter's shoulder is pain in the acromioclavicular joint due to osteolysis at the distal end of the clavicle. It is associated with the dip and press-up, and with wide-grip bench pressing. The pain is often severe at night. Treatment involves rest from the dip and press-up, and the use of a shoulder-width grip when bench pressing.

Wheels-in-line roller skating injuries

Wheels-in-line roller skating injuries can be fractures of the radial head and distal radius, fracture of the scaphoid, fracture of metacarpals and phalanges, soft tissue injuries of the hand and fractures of the leg. Death can follow a collision with a motor vehicle. Arm injuries can be prevented by wearing an appropriate splint.

Wilson's test

Wilson's test is a maneuver to determine the presence of osteochondritis dissecans of the knee in which the spine of the tibia is impinging on the lateral aspect of the medial condyle of the femur. With the patient lying supine, the test is performed by flexing the knee to 90°, internally rotating the tibia and then extending the knee slowly. The test is positive if pain is produced at about 30° of flexion.

Withdrawal syndrome
See Abstinence syndrome

Wound infection

Wound infection is characterized by cellulitis with a painful spreading erythema and by a purulent discharge from the wound. The infection is considered to be minor if there is no lymphangitis or deep tissue destruction, but major if there are painful or complete dehiscence of the fascial layers of the wound and spreading lymphangitis and cellulitis. Treatment involves the use of an appropriate antibiotic.

Wrist tendonitis

Wrist tendonitis is common in athletes, who present complaining of pain made worse by movement. There may be localized swelling. Treatment involves rest from sporting activities, splinting and non-steroidal anti-inflammatory drugs.

Y

Yergason's test

Yergason's test assesses whether pathological conditions are present in the long head of biceps in rotator cuff disorder. It is performed with the elbow flexed to 90° and the forearm pronated. The examiner grasps the wrist and resists active supination by the patient. A pathological condition is suggested by the development of pain and tenderness in the bicipital groove.

Z

Zygomatic fracture

Zygomatic fracture can occur in boxers. The suture line attachments are disrupted forming a tripod fracture, the zygoma is likely to rotate flattening the cheek and the temporomandibular joint is generally involved, so the boxer will have difficulty in opening his mouth. Treatment is conservative at first, but open reduction and internal fixation are often required.